KETTLEBELL

A Simple Guide to Learn Kettlebell Exercises

(The Ultimate Kettlebell Workouts for a Shredded Body)

Bobbie Wright

Published By Chris David

Bobbie Wright

All Rights Reserved

Kettlebell: A Simple Guide to Learn Kettlebell Exercises (The Ultimate Kettlebell Workouts for a Shredded Body)

ISBN 978-1-77485-289-7

All rights reserved. No part of this guide may be reproduced in any form without permission in writing from the publisher except in the case of brief quotations embodied in critical articles or reviews.

Legal & Disclaimer

The information contained in this book is not designed to replace or take the place of any form of medicine or professional medical advice. The information in this book has been provided for educational and entertainment purposes only.

The information contained in this book has been compiled from sources deemed reliable, and it is accurate to the best of the Author's knowledge; however, the Author cannot guarantee its accuracy and validity and cannot be held liable for any errors or omissions. Changes are periodically made to this book. You must consult your doctor or get professional medical advice before using any of the suggested remedies, techniques, or information in this book.

Upon using the information contained in this book, you agree to hold harmless the Author from and against any damages, costs, and expenses, including any legal fees potentially resulting from the application of any of the information provided by this guide. This disclaimer applies to any damages or injury caused by the use and application, whether directly or indirectly, of any advice or information presented, whether for breach of contract, tort, negligence, personal injury, criminal intent, or under any other cause of action.

You agree to accept all risks of using the information presented inside this book. You need to consult a professional medical practitioner in order to ensure you are both able and healthy enough to participate in this program.

TABLE OF CONTENTS

INTRODUCTION 1

CHAPTER 1: KETTLEBELLS - AN OVERVIEW 5

CHAPTER 2: THE BENEFITS OF KETTLEBELL TRAINING 23

CHAPTER 3: THE BACK LEGS AND GLUTES 34

CHAPTER 4: THE LOWER BODY KETTLEBELL EXERCISES 41

CHAPTER 5: EXERCISES WITH KETTLEBELLS 45

CHAPTER 6: KETTLEBELL FOUNDATION 55

CHAPTER 7: WORKOUT ROUTINE 61

CHAPTER 8: LITERATURE REVIEW 69

CHAPTER 9: KETTLEBELL TRAINING 76

CHAPTER 10: NUTRITION 86

CHAPTER 11: MANY BENEFITS OF KETTLEBELL TRAINING 91

CHAPTER 12: INTERMEDIATE KETTLEBELL EXERCISES 112

CHAPTER 13: KETTLEBELLS BEGINNER'S WORKOUT 135

CHAPTER 14: GUIDELINES FOR STRUCTURED WORKOUTS 146

CHAPTER 15: SOLUTIONS COMMON MISTAKES TO AVOID KETTLEBELL EXERCISES 162

CHAPTER 16: WHAT IS KETTLEBELL TRAINING? 165

CHAPTER 17: 30- DAYS OF KETTLEBELL WOD EXERCISES 174

CONCLUSION 181

Introduction

Kettlebells were used since the beginning of the 1800s when Russian powerful men wore kettlebells in a variety of dimensions and forms. It's interesting to notice in looking at photographs from the beginning of these powerful men that their bodies were more athletic and proportional to the physiques we now think of as bodybuilding. Although bodybuilding began in the 1940s, it really began to take off in the 1980s due to the widespread use of machines that enabled gym owners to bring more people into their gyms without the need for training or supervision being needed. Machines confine you to a certain direction of motion. This frees your stabilising muscles from having to perform any part of the work required by machines and exposes the possibility of injury trying to control weight within a plane of movement that you've not developed.

Unfortunately, this has led to the strength training ignoring its purpose to focus on Mirror muscles i.e. chest and the biceps.

Isolation was the new word for training. It works well to build the specific muscles being isolated, but isn't helping the body perform effectively as a whole. In the last five years we've seen a revival of functional training like Crossfit using Olympic lifts as well as tyre flips, kettlebells and exercises that use body weight.

There's a lot to say about the importance of a minimalist approach to training and doing anything more than you need to is a waste of time and energy. Through kettlebell's compound movement it is possible to engage several muscle groups simultaneously which increases the calories burnand improving the body's capacity to work together, and achieve more in a shorter amount of time. The majority of exercise sessions are made up of three or two exercises, and can be completed in less than 30 minutes. The best part is that the rhythm that is created by kettlebells is what makes them enjoyable and addicting.

The use of kettlebells makes it simpler to complete your exercise routine and workout since you don't have to consider the equipment that will work what muscle group, and the size or weight you'll need to choose to get a exercise. You don't need to determine the days that you should be doing cardio and when you should work on strength as kettlebells are a great way to combine strength and cardio training. The majority of kettlebell workouts target your posterior chain. It is incredibly beneficial, not just in terms of athletic performance, but as well to improve position and back stability. Back pain in the lower back is usually caused by weak glutes which can cause muscles in the erector spinal region to overcompensate and stiff hip muscles (caused due to working in office chairs for the entire day) that cause back pain because they cause the pelvis to tilt inwards. The exercise of kettlebells can strengthen the gluteal muscles, which help alleviate the erector spine muscles. It also increases hip flexor flexibility. This helps to reduce pelvic tilt and lower back pain.

Certain kettlebell exercises help build your power-endurance, the capacity to sustain rapid muscle contractions for a long period of time. Examples of these are the snatch, and explosively executed swings or squats. While both strength and power are important qualities to possess Power-endurance is typically what determines the winner of sporting events. Training for power-endurance is also great to lose fat and improve your conditioning.

Chapter 1: Kettlebells - An Overview

What is a KELLELL?

If you think of the shape of a cannonball, with handles attached to the top, that's exactly what kettlebells look like. They are usually made of either cast iron or steel and their ancestors can be traced to Russian girya. The girya's beginnings originate in the 18th century, when the girya was utilized to measure the crops. In the 19th century, similar weights were also being utilized by circus strongmen to show their the strength. In the latter part of the 19th century, kettlebells came into the arena of recreational and competitive strength athletics. In 1885, the sport of girevoy was born, a kind of lifting kettlebells for competition. In the 20th century, kettlebells were recognized worldwide and the English name "kettle bell" was used.

BALLISTIC TRAINING

Kettlebells are gaining popularity on the main market due to their versatility and effectiveness as a tool for full-body fitness. The kettlebell exercises are known as ballistic and power exercise. To better understand the ballistics of training completely, it is necessary to know the power formula.

Force + Velocity = Power

To simplify Power x Speed = Power

In terms of velocity, we refer to the speed at the speed at which a weight such as kettlebells, travels and the direction it's traveling in. The force that is exerted by the kettlebell is a measure of the strength you're applying to move the kettlebell and, most importantly, to accelerate the kettlebell.

Speed and strength are in opposition to one another in this manner. The heavier an item is the more slow it will move, however more strength is needed in order to get it moving. The lighter the object the more quickly it'll move, however the lesser strength it requires in order to get it moving. This means it's impossible to train for maximal speed and strength simultaneously. The best way to train for most effective results is to work at the middle of the twoat around 30%-80 percent of your own one-rep max weight.

One-rep maximum is the maximum amount you are able to lift during one workout for example, an exercise like a bench press or dead lift. If you are able to lift 100 pounds, the ideal mid-point would be a kettlebell weighing 30 to 80 pounds to train ballistic. When speed and strength collide at the mid-point that you can train more efficiently and effectively. You're lifting as much weight as you can in as fast as you can without speed or strength being affected by being heavy and slow or being too light and quick.

BENEFITS of BALLISTIC Training Using KETTLEBELLS

Burning fat: Running has for a long time been touted as the ideal exercise to lose fat and gain lean. Kettlebells have thrown that notion off the table. According to the

American Council on Exercise (ACE) conducted a study which showed that, for one minute of using kettlebells, you can lose 20 calories. (No author. 2019September 1,). This would translate to a 400-calorie burn within a 20-minute time. To burn off 400 calories within twenty minutes running you'd have be running at a speed of six minutes for every mile.

The Post Burn The After Burn of kettlebell exercise results in an excessive post-exercise oxygen consumption (EPEOC). In simple terms, it boosts the calorie burn after exercise, which increases the effectiveness of the exercise. The greater the amount of burning calories and the longer the impact persists as well, the more fat will burn following your exercise.

Lang-term Calorie Burn Training using kettlebells will increase the amount of lean muscle mass you have. Muscles require greater calories than fat to stay functioning. The greater the muscle mass you have the higher the amount of calories you'll burn off at any time even when you are relaxing.

Get rid of the gym Do not put off getting in shape since you don't want join a gym. You can become fit, strong and lean without leaving your home; all you require is kettlebells.

Reduce space and money Comparatively to other equipment for home use, kettlebells are comparatively affordable in the long run. It's not necessary to start with a complete set of various sizes. All you need is a kettlebell that is the right weight and you're good to go to start.

Strong, Lean, Mean Machine: Kettlebells will help you increase your muscle mass However, don't get intimidated. It's not likely that you'll lose your feminine appeal due to big male muscles. Kettlebells are a great way to build muscles that are lean. This will help you achieve that toned and shapely physique you've always wanted and boost your strength and strength without the weight.

Strength and Cardio: Kettlebell exercises mix the benefits of cardiovascular exercise from fast-paced moves with the strength building benefits that comes from using weights. It is possible to achieve two distinct objectives in your training with just one exercise which makes it more efficient and efficient.

Fitness for Functional Strength using kettlebells helps develop what's called functional strength. Utilizing different muscles groups in your body, the workout builds strength needed for everyday tasks that make you stronger, as well as less prone to injuries.

Five-in-One Workout - Training with kettlebells does more than just boost the strength and speed. You'll also increase strength, endurance and stability.

All-in-One Training: Stop doing a lot of different exercises that concentrate on just one muscles at a. The training sessions you take will target various muscles simultaneously and will give you a complete body workout all in one session.

From the Right To the Core Kettlebells have a great effect in building your core strength. The muscles in your core help stabilize your body and provide support. The strength of your core is vital for good posture, ease of movement, and to avoid injury while doing everyday tasks.

Control: Training with kettlebells usually involves a variety of exercises and develops consciousness of the body. It is the connection that you have between your brain and muscles as well as your focus will increase, leading to general better coordination.

Alternative Cardio: You're mixing strength and speed training which makes kettlebells an effective substitute for traditional cardio-based exercises. If you're seeking a way to get off the treadmill however, you still want to improve your cardiovascular health metabolism, improve your fitness level, and reduce fat, then kettlebells could be the solution you require.

Strengthening the hips: The kettlebell swing is among the most well-known and efficient kettlebell exercises. It can help train your hips to increase power and speed. A greater amount of power in your hips can lead to better stability, and lower risks of injuries.

Flexibility and mobility: Kettlebell training is multi planar. It is about managing the force you are applying to the movements, tongue, as well as your range. With time, your limits will grow and you will have a greater and more varied range of motion, as well as greater flexibility.

Posture is perfect: Kettlebells strengthen your hamstrings and gluteal muscles. They also strengthen your pelvic and hip muscles trapezius and lower back muscles shoulder, neck, and trapezius muscles. While simultaneously strengthening the strength of all these muscles, and your core is a great way to develop an excellent musculoskeletal foundation.

Find a grip: Kettlebell training develops a solid, sturdy grip by training your fingers, wrists and your forearm. It is time to stop needing help to open containers.

Evening on the Field: A majority of people have a dominant part of their body which is stronger in comparison to the opposite. Kettlebell exercises can help you identify areas in need of improvement as well as even out the strengths differences within your body.

Joint health: Kettlebell exercise helps in increasing joint strength, stability mobility, flexibility, and eventually increasing the range of motion.

Keep it simple Kettlebells are a simple. There is no need for a wide range of fitness equipment or perform a lot of complex exercises. Kettlebells are also extremely mobile, making them easy to pack into your car to ensure you can workout anytime you're bored anywhere you happen to be. If there's a thing that will keep you focused on your fitness routine is not having any excuse to not work out.

Are KETTLEBELLS for you?

People who are able to consider giving kettlebells a go are:

Anyone looking to reap the benefits that exercising with kettlebells brings

Anyone who wants to exercise in the privacy and comfort in the privacy of their home

Anyone who would like to alter their fitness regimen or experiment with an entirely new exercise routine which incorporates exercises that have been tested to be efficient

Back injuries sufferers who wish to build muscle and strengthen their bodies, but don't want to put extra or unnecessary stress on their spine.

Athletes looking to increase their fitness and overall performance in their chosen discipline.

THE (VERY very few) SIDES DOWNSIDES

Like everything else in life, kettlebells are a must. They come with positive points as well as there are some disadvantages, too.

Cost: Although they might not cost a fortune however, high-quality kettlebells require an investment in money. The good thing is that you can start by purchasing just one, and then buy more as you advance.

Form and injury Movements and exercises are fluid, they work in multiple directions, utilize numerous muscles simultaneously and require stability, balance and strength. Proper form is crucial to avoid injury, which is why it is important to study and practice regularly and master your form before attempting to build strength.

Space: Kettlebells can be small and compact when compared to larger gym equipment for home use, however they are still a big burden. You must find a secure, safe, and out of the way place to store your bells so that you don't fall over them. It's not ideal to put your toe in an iron cannonball cast in cast; trust me when I say it won't be amusing!

In the majority of cases, kettlebells aren't adjustable. You'll need to add more kettlebells to your collection or replace the kettlebells that you do not require with more modern heavy kettlebells. Kettlebells will cost you over time , to increase your fitness and not a one-time price at the beginning. The good thing is that the price isn't excessive with every improvement, and your health and body is worth investing in.

KETTLEBELLS DUMBBELLS VS KETTLEBELLS BATTLE ROYALE

Both dumbbells and kettlebells have "battled" for fame and preferential treatment over one another for many years. What's the difference? which one is the winner of the best training device?

Weight Loss

Winner: Kettlebells

The traditional strength training with dumbbells can aid in weight loss, however it's not the most effective in this regard and takes longer than kettlebells.

Bulk Vs Lean

Winner: Kettlebells

They isolate muscle groups and are commonly employed to build bulk muscles. Kettlebells make use of fluid movements along with cardio and resistance training to build muscles for a slimmer and toned look.

Friendly for beginners

Winner: Dumbbells

Exercises with dumbbells are easier and less paced for novices to weight and strength training. Kettlebells may require some adjustment and practice before using the correct posture.

Incremental Growth

Winner: Dumbbells

Kettlebells are sold in fixed sizes. That means kettlebells are sold with increments of between 9 to 18 pounds. They aren't tiny increments that can be challenges when it comes to increasing the weight of your kettlebell. Dumbbells provide increments of between 1 and 2 pounds. at a given time, allowing the possibility of increasing weight in smaller, less manageable increments.

Balance

Winner: Draw

When using kettlebells, the weight is not balanced when compared to dumbbells. It may appear to be an issue, but it's not necessarily a negative thing. When using kettlebells, all the weight rests on the base of the hand, which makes them difficult to use. This helps improve the balance and coordination of the user and focusing more muscles. Off-balance-weights offer a variety of kinds of exercises and grips that make them more effective and adaptable.

Dumbbells on their own, have greater stability and balance. They are more convenient to use due to the more balanced weights as well as requiring less coordination. The tussle is an end in a draw since each works in different ways according to the goals you have set.

Grip

Winner: Kettlebells

The grip that kettlebells use and dumbbells is radically different. They only have one type of grip, while kettlebells have an array of grip options with different angles. They help develop an even more solid grip than dumbbells due to this different grip style and the imbalanced characteristics of weight.

Handle Smoothly

Winner: Draw

Handles of kettlebells are more smooth than the dumbbells' bars. The dumbbells must offer users a smooth surface to provide a more comfortable grip, with a non-slip surface. Kettlebells should feature a smooth, rounded handle to ensure that they move freely and easily within your hands. Each handle has its own function for the exercise they were designed for, and this fight comes to a close.

Functional Strength

Winner: Kettlebells

The dumbbells are targeted at specific areas and muscle groups with restricted, non-functional movements. Kettlebells offer a greater variety of exercises that target a variety of muscles groups and replicate the daily routine. This improves the fitness you can achieve in your everyday life.

Cardio

Winner: Kettlebells

Do not be surprised if dumbbells leave you huffing and puffing out of exhaustion when you're using weights that are that are heavy enough to test your muscles to the limit. The drawback is that with all that sweating and breathing this isn't an aerobic workout. Kettlebells make use of exercises that offer an exercise that is cardio-based and a resistance training exercise simultaneously.

Mixing It Up

Winner: Kettlebells

The dumbbells aren't as versatile and simple to throw into a workout routine like kettlebells. If you're tired of your routine fitness routine, you can add kettlebell exercises to mix things up a little. Not only will it help to eliminate boredom, you'll find new muscles to exercise, strengthen and strengthen.

Time

Winner: Kettlebells

The dumbbell is a tried and tested method to build strength, but this is where their value is over. The strength training using dumbbells needs an increased amount of time to exercise each muscle group individually. Additionally, you must incorporate cardio into your workout routine. Kettlebells can save you time by providing a fast whole-body fitness and cardio exercise in one session.

Affordable

Winner: Dumbbells

Kettle bells might not be an investment that is costly for your fitness and health However, they have a price. Dumbbells reduce expenses by using one bar on which you can put various weight plates that can be interchanged. The cost per pound of dumbbells tends to be lower than kettlebells however both are excellent choices to train at home, and both are worthy of the investment.

Chapter 2: The benefits Of Kettlebell Training

There are numerous benefits that you can reap when you do kettlebell exercises. The most important thing to remember is that kettlebell workouts provide an unique mix of benefits from cardiovascular exercises and strength. Like we said earlier, the kettlebell training is more unique and is a lot like the shape of a cannonball that has the handle attached. It is a great way to increase your endurance, strength, agility, improve endurance and balance, while also helping burning fat.

Kettlebell exercises usually include many different swings and lifts. The best part is that the tool is very adaptable and can be utilized to do a wide range of training activities that are intense. If you are looking for a system that is a mix of cardio and strength, kettlebells are the best choice to create exercises that are not only efficient, but also time-efficient.

If you're considering whether to swap out your traditional dumbbells in favor of something that's going to be worthwhile Here are some of the advantages that you shouldn't skip when choosing kettlebells for training.

1. Improve Your Form

One of the most important aspects that separate kettlebells from D is the offset of the weight. This is because it's center of gravity for kettlebells is approximately 6-8 inches from your hand when you grip the handle. This is why it is very difficult to manage.

This is why, for every exercise you take on, from traditional strength exercises to more challenging kettlebell workouts like swings will require an exact form and more stimulation of the muscles that you can get with a dumbbells.

Consider the overhead press. In this scenario one of the most enjoyable things about dumbbells is that many people are content to push until they have their elbows bent to an angle that is right. But, with kettlebells it is the opposite.

Our instinct is to press to secure. This is due to the offset load functions as a counterweight which can play a crucial role in pulling shoulders back.

Also, the kettlebell is an important component in assisting you to complete each exercise perfectly and in a perfect way. If, however, you are unable to accomplish something, such as find yourself arching your back or turning to one side as you try to finish the exercise and you end up twisting to one side, then you realize that your technique is not working properly.

If you do squats with the kettlebell behind your body This will cause you to recline, which increases the efficiency of your squat squat a lot. This paves your way to move on to more challenging exercises as you gain strength.

2. Enhances Core Strength

If you push an overhead kettlebell and over your head, you're just making your back and ribs to flare. This means you must to keep your core in place as tight as you can to maintain your posture. If you are taking an exercise, it is crucial to strengthen your core in order to prevent that your spine from turning in the lower part of the

actions. So, for every exercise you can be sure that you can expect your core to be working harder in the hopes for stabilizing the body and making sure that your safety is the first priority.

3. Enhance the athleticism

If you're an athlete one of the main advantages of using kettlebells as part of your training routine is that you build up grip strength. This is due to the handle of the kettlebell along with the load being displaced needs your fingers, hands, and forearms to ensure complete control compared to dumbbells.

Many manufacturers favor large handlesfor their products, one aspect you must be aware of is that when you choose the handle that is narrower that you make it much easier to complete complicated moves. This can increase your options for training.

Because grip strength is higher than in many activities, as well as increasing general strength, kettlebells have the possibility of increasing your endurance in the cardiovascular department. The kettlebell workouts often involve the entire body, and

exercises like the press clean and snatch require lifting weights from the floor and over the head. This makes sure that muscles throughout the body are working effectively and create an enormous strain of the cardiovascular system. In the end, many athletes make kettlebells as an integral part of their training programs.

4. Easy Accessibility

Like exercises bands as well as suspension trainers kettlebells are also very portable and are easy to take along on your travels. They do not be a nuisance in your car the way dumbbells do. They won't be odd when you take along to the shore with you.

Furthermore unlike the dumbbell there is only one kettlebell in order to get a good exercise. It is because using just one kettlebell, you will be able to participate in many exercises, in contrast to the dumbbell which is why you require a couple of choices of them for your routine workouts.

If you plan on exercising your entire body, it is possible to carry two kettlebells. It is true that if you only have one kettlebell, you can use it.

the corner of your bedroom or even the back in your automobile, you'll probably likely have a gym in the back of your car or in the corner of your room.

5. Lowers Body Fat

Many people want to shed some pounds, and weight loss is among their main fitness objectives. The benefit of kettlebell-training is it allows you to do this effortlessly. The reason behind this is kettlebell training incorporates numerous intense workouts that enable your body to burn as many calories as it is possible.

Although many weight loss programs require a lot of time and effort to reach the ideal weight and body shape and then get boring after a while the kettlebell workout is different. It is because it provides an exciting alternative to regular exercise routine because it keeps you on track and increase the rate of your metabolism.

It is strongly suggested that if you plan to shed weight through kettlebell training, that you incorporate high repetition compound workout into every session. The exercises you can do include kettlebell swings, reverse lunges or shoulder presses. Most important is to make sure that you don't have any time to rest between each exercise.

6. Improves Posture

One of the problems that happens to our bodies is, as we get older our posture is affected. But the good news is that it is possible to be sure that you can reduce the consequences of aging by including kettlebells into your exercise routine. It is due to the fact that, according to studies, there's evidence that shows that kettlebells are effective in reducing the effects of aging.

Exercises can help improve posture and counteract the effects of our contemporary lifestyles.

When working out it's typical for the muscles of the postural region not to get attention. With kettlebells you will notice improvements faster and better your posture. Are you aware of why this is so important? A better posture makes you appear slimmer and improves self-esteem as well as confidence.

7. Cheap

Kettlebells can be a good value. If you purchase the best kettlebell you can rest assured that they will last for a long time and you won't have to pay the expense of replacing them often.

For the majority of beginners, an individual kettlebell constructed from solid steel can last for a long time. Furthermore, kettlebell exercises do not require you to be in special footwear as with other exercises, which will help you are able to save money you could have spending on a high-priced pair of exercise shoes.

8. Gaining Strength without Bulk

Do you realize that the majority of women who exercise share an innate desire to build their strength, without having an appearance that is as bulky as the male bodybuilder? With kettlebells the goal is not to build strength of the muscles but to improve strength , without being bulky.

This is because when you add kettlebell exercises into your fitness program, you're using full body functional exercises. These exercises play a crucial function in simultaneously targeting a variety of muscles throughout the body. If you have any specific requirements, it is recommended to speak with your trainer to ensure they can develop exercises that satisfy these needs.

9. User-friendly

Contrary to dumbbells which carry the potential to strain your arms or other workouts that can put the risk of injury kettlebells are extremely easy to use. It is because they don't force the muscles of the body too much. They are more relaxed.

The weights are able to rest comfortably on your forearms, without weighing them down or creating fatigue. This is why women like kettlebells to other exercises that require weight.

10. Quick Workout

The majority of us don't have the time to register and go to the gym. However, this doesn't mean that there aren't exercises to aid in keeping your body in top shape. Kettlebell exercises are great for you and you can practice them from the comfort of your office, home or at any other location you feel comfortable in.

Kettlebells work on a variety of muscles throughout the body, and that means you don't have to devote so much time with other workouts which only focus on only one part of your body at an time. This is why kettlebells are the ideal choice for people with busy schedules, like mothers. And the best part is, you can do these exercises without supervision.

Chapter 3: The Back Legs and Glutes

This chapter will review of the various exercises that focus on the lower body as well as the back, as well as the various advantages that can be gained through these exercises by using kettlebells. There are a lot of exercises that target the back and legs in kettlebells, but a lot are obliterated by the fact that a few have a significant impact on other muscle groups, including the core muscles as well as the arms.

When doing these workouts the reason that these muscles are affected is due to the fact that (especially in arm muscles) it is because they're the ones that first hold the weight, or shift the weight to them in a flash during the exercise. Let's start with a workout.

1. The Kettlebell Clean

Group of muscles to target: Legs, the Glutes, and Back

Walkthrough This can be a workout that you can do in its entirety, however it is also an essential step to master in transition. It's one of the classic girevoy movesand, when performed during transition, it is an excellent method to initiate exercises that provide you with a complete fitness routine for your body. Although it's been practiced with a barbell during traditional bodybuilding for a long time but the distinctiveness of kettlebell cleans has meant that more experienced body builders use this specific exercise to supplement their bar training workouts. The advantages of performing kettlebell cleans are more effective and powerful technique that is fairly easy to master and produces impressive results.

To clean the kettlebell first, put the kettlebell on your feet. The weight should be lifted upwards with your shoulders shrugging as you pull yourself and your kettlebell toward your shoulder while doing this. The bell should be resting on your forearm, which is tucked into your body using your hands on your chest, in what's called the "rack" position. The weight should be brought back to the floor for one repetition.

As was mentioned previously as a must technique to learn not just for the purpose of transition but also because it will aid in building your legs and lower back.

2. It is the Kettlebell Goblet Squat

It is among the most effective exercises for the lower body that you can perform with kettlebells and is among the best commonly used exercises available. Much like the standard squat exercise, this one is a little different which make this exercise that is unique to kettlebells.

Muscle group to target: The glutes, legs, and the back

Walkthrough: Since it is an altered version of the squat the ideal position to begin in is standing straight with your feet separated by a shoulder and holding the kettlebell near your chest. Squat back down, pushing your hips forward while pushing your heels towards the ground until your hips are at a 90-degree angle or higher in relation to the ground. Reverse to your standing position for one repetition.

As with all conventional exercises, there is the risk of serious damage to your spine and lower back when this exercise isn't performed in a safe manner and in a correct posture. Keep this in mind and ensure that while performing the exercise, your spine is in a straight position. This will not only assist you to prevent injury, but it will also aid in building core strength and stability.

3. Lateral Lunge Passes

Target muscle group: Legs, Back, Glutes

The walkthrough below explains how lateral lunges are one of the lesser-known exercises available, but they're very important to lower body exercises because they target in slightly different muscles in the lower part of the body as opposed to traditional lunges. This intriguing alternative to the conventional lunge lateral is certainly something that can add some variety to a routine workout. It's something more like a crossfit type exercise rather than a fluid-style exercise, and it is very easy to master it is to master.

Start by standing up straight, your feet positioned by a shoulder. While holding the kettlebell with your left hand, move it to your left, making sure you have your spine straight, and that the hips are moved slightly forward. As you lunge to your left, you should swing the kettlebell left in the same direction as the lunge. Pass it to your left hand when the kettle reaches the halfway point. Repeat the movement and pass it from right to left, this time, and count the entire procedure as one rep.

Through these lateral lunge runs even though they are targeted at the lower part of the body they're also efficient in building muscle strength in the shoulders and arms since the muscles involved are also activated by swinging the kettlebell side to the other side.

4. This is the Kettlebell Deadlift.

Target muscle group: Legs, Glutes, Back

A walkthrough of the traditional deadlift is a common element in all workout routines and barbells are among the top essential items of equipment. The exercise has proven to be beneficial for strengthening the lower back, and is executed correctly. It's also an crucial exercise when it comes to core and leg strength because it not only strengthens the lower back, but it also helps shape and mold the glutes and legs.

In this particular exercise you should forget about the barbell and take out the kettlebell, because this exercise is able to be done far more efficiently with kettlebells and will yield the same , if not better results.

To do the kettlebell deadlift first place the kettlebell on your ground between your toes. With the back straight squat low and hold the kettlebell using both hands. While keeping your muscles aligned and the glutes tight place your heels on the ground. Gradually rise into a standing position and then lift the weight behind your. Similar to traditional deadlifts using barbells, make sure to maintain your proper posture while you perform the movements, since this exercise could cause back injuries if not done correctly.

5. It is the Two Arm Kettlebell Row

Muscle group of interest: Back

Walkthrough: When people think of rowing usually, they imagine a rowing machine at your gym or going to a lake or pond in a boat and rowing across the ocean expanse. Some people think of rowing as something that could be performed in waters, but could also be performed in the gym using an exercise bar or dumbbell along with a few weights. There is another method to perform this awesome exercise and that is with kettlebells.

The weights provide a fascinating variation to the exercise and they can more than just increase the strength of your lower and upper back. In addition to the benefits for your arms the kettlebell row may be beneficial to your core and chest when executed correctly, which makes it an exercise that is among the best and complete back exercises available.

Begin by taking two kettlebells , and put them in front of both feet. Turn your body over while bent your knees slightly while maintaining the back in a straight position. Take both kettlebells and push them toward your stomach while keeping your elbows near to your body while doing this. Lower the weight until you've completed one repetition.

This type of exercise is perfect to build arm and shoulder strength and the posture it demands ensures ample stabilization and strength are as well developed if performed right.

Chapter 4: The Lower Body

Kettlebell Exercises

Kettlebell Squat (Thighs)
Hold the kettlebell at chest height using both hands, keeping your elbows in a

tucked-in position and your hands close to your body.

The feet of your feet must be slightly wider than shoulder width apart and your toes should be slightly pointing toward the outside.

Intensify your abs and ensure that your lower back is straight. This is the starting posture of the workout.

Begin to bend your knees gradually and then bring your hips back to the ground, then lower your legs until you reach the point where your thighs are a less than parallel to the ground. When you're done take a deep breath and exhale.

- Restore yourself to your original or starting posture by pushing the hips forward and pressing your heels. When you're done exhale. This is 1 rep.

- Perform 8-12 reps for each set.

The Deadlift of a Kettlebell with a One-Legged Leg (Hamstrings)

Begin with standing up on one foot with a kettlebell on one hand and the other hand is on the opposite end of the leg the leg you're standing on.

- While standing with your leg bent slightly then perform a stiff-legged deadlift by stretching the opposite leg toward your back while you bend your hips. Extending your other leg will help keep your body in balance during the exercise.

- Keep bringing down the kettlebell until the upper part of your body is almost in line with the floor.

- Repeat the move in reverse and then return to the beginning position to complete one rep.

Do between 8 and 12 repetitions per set.

Kettlebell Bulgarian Split Squat (Thighs and Glutes)

If you place one foot on the top of a container or bench and hold a kettle bell on each side of each.

If you are putting your weight on the heels of your front leg, and bringing your chest forward then move your legs until your knee which is up on the platform or box behind you touches the floor. Be sure that the knee of your front leg doesn't extend beyond the toes to limit the risk for knee injuries.

Return to your original position for 1 rep. Perform 8-12 reps for each set for each leg.

Chapter 5: Exercises with Kettlebells

10 Kettlebell Exercises

Kettlebells have gained a lot of attention because it has been proven to be beneficial to the cardio, strength, and flexibility training. There are a variety of sizes of kettlebells and methods that an individual must master to meet their goals. It is generally recommended that women start with weights of 8-16 kg and men should begin with 16-32 kg. But, the amount of sets and reps is dependent on the fitness level required. Thanks to technology, you are able to see how to execute these moves properly! Furthermore, there are many kinds of kettlebell exercises that will be discussed in depth in the following article:

Russian Kettlebell Swing: This exercise is suitable for beginners and targets the shoulders, back as well as the legs and hips. To ensure a precise kettlebell swings, your posture is to be straight while in a standing in a position that is slightly larger than the hip distance. After the posture has been established then hold your kettlebell's handle using both hands, keeping the palms facing up and the arms forward of the body. Make sure to bend slightly at the knee, then drive the hips forward while dropping the body. It is crucial to ensure that the body isn't too high. After that, using an fluid motion, with the core and glutes engaged and accelerating your hips forward while lifting the kettlebell. Additionally it is crucial to ensure that the movement does not originate from the arm , but rather from the hips as the body is returned to standing. The motion should be continued for between 12 and 15 reps, while slowly lifting the weight to the knees. In addition, because this exercise is intended for beginners the weight of the kettlebell must be sufficient to avoid injuries. This video provides an example.

Kettlebell Figure 8: This exercise is recommended for intermediate levels and is focused on the back, arms, and abs of the individual. To perform it correctly, it is essential to keep your back straight and the chest elevated while keeping your legs slightly more than the hip-width distance. The ideal position is dropping the body to the quarter-squat posture. Many people don't understand the correct position, and maintain the posture in the standing squat. After establishing the correct position you can hold the kettlebell using the left hand, then swing it to along the side of the leg and then return to the middle of your legs. Then repeat the exercise with your right hand, and continue to swing the kettlebell. In this sequence it is crucial to ensure that the switch from left hand to right is completed in the middle. This video shows an example.

Kettlebell Goblet squat: It is the most popular type of swingthat targets the back, legs, and glutes. This kind of squat is designed intended for intermediate level that requires straight posture. The kettlebell should be held close to the chest using both hands and the elbows near to the body. Start squatting through driving your heels towards the ground and then pushing the hips forward until your thighs are level with the ground or below. It is recommended to continue this for 15 to 20 repetitions. Many people are able to do this easily and want to do more reps, without being concerned about posture. But, the emphasis should be on quality of the swing rather than the amount of swing. The example of this is in the video .

Kettlebell High Pull: This exercise is focused on glutes, shoulders, arms and the legs. It is a good exercise for intermediate levels and novices are not advised to begin with it. For proper technique it is recommended to keep the kettlebell on the ground between the legs. Toes and legs should be positioned 45 degrees, with feet a little wider than shoulder width apart. Start squatting and keep the core in place. The kettlebell's handle is to be controlled with just one hand. Next, using the force from the hips and heels, push to stand by pulling the kettlebell to the upward direction while the elbow pushes it upwards. Following this, lower to the ground and switch arms. The goal should be 10-12 for each arm. The example from this clip.

Kettlebell Free: This workout is designed for advanced levels and those who are new to the sport are advised not to attempt this for the first time. Because it's intense intensity, it could result in injury for those who have not been skilled. It concentrates on the legs, butts, and back. This is the reason people with back injuries should not be doing it. For the purpose of doing the exercise properly you must begin the exercise in an upwards with the feet. The shoulders should be slack, pulling the body and the 'bell upwards towards the shoulder. The kettlebell should be in"rack" position "rack" position, which is resting on your forearm, that is resting near to the body. Your fist should be in your chest. Then, the exercise should be repeated for 10 repetitions, while lifting the kettlebell to the floor. Furthermore kettlebell clean is thought to be to be one of the most effective exercises since it helps increase shoulder strength and strengthen the core strength. It also has a beneficial training effect when it is performed for a prolonged period. An example is shown in this video.

Single-Arm Kettlebell Split Jerk: It's crucial to make sure that the knees are able to support pressure as the main purpose of the exercise is the chest, shoulders, back and legs. If the position isn't correct, it could cause injury to the legs and back. So, it's best suitable for advanced levels. Begin with cleaning the kettlebell until the shoulder and then finishing it with the front facing palm. Then, push the kettlebell upwards in a bent in the split jerk movement slowly. Then return to a standing and ensure that the your kettlebell overhead and afterwards lower the kettlebell. Repeat the exercise for between 4 and 6 on each side for those who are doing it for this first time. An example can be found in this video.

Two-Arm Kettlebell Military Press: This is the most advanced form of kettlebell exercise that can be classified as a high intensity workout since it involves two kettlebells. It can help increase strength, strength and flexibility in the body. It works with both small and large muscles. Additionally, it produces force from the core upwards towards the object that it is trying to manage. The emphasis is on the arms, shoulders, and the back in the back of our body. Then, to begin the exercise keep the kettlebells on the rack and wash them until they are in an "rack" place. It is crucial to make sure that the kettlebells' grip are strong. After that, lift the kettlebells upwards position while leaning forward towards the waist until the weights are placed on the back of your head. The kettlebells should be returned to the shoulder and continue this for 10-20 reps. In this workout, it is important to choose the correct kettlebell size so that you do not cause any injuries to your hands. The example is shown in the video.

Kettlebell Push-Up and Row This exercise is of a higher level and requires a push-up posture. It targets the back, chest as well as the arms. It is crucial to get the proper posture. In the position of a push-up you should hold the kettlebell with the right hand and do an exercise called a push-up. When you reach the top, raise the right elbow while squeezing the shoulder blades and the weight placed about 6 inches from the body. When you've done it correctly then return to the starting position and repeat in 5-8 repetitions using both arms. Many people make mistakes in getting the correct posture, making it challenging to do the push up correctly. A good example can be seen found in the following video.

Kettlebell Windmill Kettlebell Windmill is an advanced exercise that targets the shoulders, back abs, oblique's and hips. To perform this exercise correctly you need to place a kettlebell the front of the lead foot, wash the kettlebell, then push it up using the opposite hand. Clean the kettlebell toward shoulder by stretching the hips and legs while you pull the kettlebell to the shoulders. Then, turn your wrist until the palm is facing toward the front. Then, press it up by extensing the elbow. In order to keep the kettlebell locked in all times and push the butt away toward the kettlebell locked out. The feet should be turned out at 45 degrees to the arm holding the kettlebell that is locked out. The hips should be bent towards one direction, extending the butt in, slowly lean forward until the floor is completely covered with hands free of. One of the most common mistakes the majority of people make when doing the exercise is to not maintain the position that can be compared to a triangular poses or keep the body in control of their body. An example is shown on this clip.

Side Step Kettlebell Swing This exercise is suitable for intermediate and advanced levels, based on the weight of kettlebell. The primary targets for the swing are glutes, legs and back of the body, and back. In the first step, hold the kettlebell using both of the hands , and begin with an easy two-handed swing. Then, bring the legs in as the bell drops between them, then step left foot towards the left. Then after the bell is raised then bring the left foot towards the right. Repeat for 10 to 15 reps. Then, use the left foot to complete the exercise. The most frequent mistake that many make is not paying attention to the posture of their legs that must be in close proximity in order to complete the exercise. An example is shown on this clip.

Chapter 6: Kettlebell Foundation

They might not appear like many things, but they are an all-in-one gym. You've probably noticed that kettlebells feature a distinctive style that distinguishes them from other equipment for training out there. A kettlebell is a forged iron weight which appears similar to a ball from a cannon however, it has an attached handle. What makes this device so effective is the shape of the handle that allows the central weight in the kettlebell to extend out beyond the hand. This makes it an ideal device for ballsy movements like swings. Ballistic exercises are a fantastic choice since they incorporate the elements of strength, cardio and flexibility in one amazing exercise.

The ballistic movement also allows you to improve your functional fitness that mimics the actions we do in our daily lives like clearing snow.

Two main functions of kettlebells:

(1) The development of functional fitness

(2) Specially designed training for competitions with kettlebells

In this book, we'll focus on only exercises that are functional and will get rid of body fat as you build muscle bulking you up, and improving your fitness.

Learning To Know Your Kettlebell

Kettlebells are either adjustable or fixed load. Of course, kettlebells that are fixed load are more efficient and easy to use since there is no need to switch resistances in between moves.

The handle of the kettlebell is the element of the apparatus that you are most likely to come into contact with. The kettlebell handle can be extremely smooth to very rough. You'll want one that's not too smooth, nor too rough, yet will allow for a secure grip when your hands sweat.

The unique design that the kettlebell has makes it an ideal choice for a variety of exercises. The design of the weight as well as the space between it and the ball allows swinging, catch and release motions. It also permits the weight to rest directly on the arm, which gives more leverage. This allows for a an even alignment between the arm and hand also helps to increase the endurance of the arm muscles during the workout.

The kettlebells you will find in your gym are typically between 8 kg (18 pounds) to 48kg (106 pounds). The average male should begin with a 16kg (35 pounds) bell, and the majority of women begin their working out with an 8kg (18 pounds) bell.

Tips for Clothing

Beware of wearing loose clothes that could become caught in the kettlebell when doing the swings. It is also important to be wary of the slick designs and logos on your clothes that will cause you to sweat and make it harder for you to hold your hands at your side.

Don't wear clothes that are too tight. It is not a good idea for your forefinger or thumb to be caught in the baggy portion of your crotch while you're performing swing-type actions. A tight fitting pair of shorts is an excellent idea.

Safety

Make sure there is an area of at least one square one meter (3.3 sq. feet) surrounding you when you're using kettlebells.

If you're caught in the middle of the rep, do not try to get the rep back by relocating away from the area and let gravity work its magic.

If you can, you should use chalk to keep you hands from turning slippery.

A towel is handy to remove sweat.

Drink plenty of water throughout your workout.

Wear wristbands for protection from the wrists from chaffing and forearms.

Wear shoes with sturdy flat soles.

Always raise or lower the kettlebell with control (bend as you lower!)

Kettlebell Movement Technique

The majority of kettlebell exercises involve at least two of these grips

Finger hook grip

Hand grip for insertion

A palm up grip is formed by inserting your middle finger into your kettlebell's middle. Put the index finger underneath the thumb and create an a hook for the finger.

It is important to avoid these common grip errors:

Too tight grip on the handle

Letting the handle hang too loosely

Only holding with the fingertips

Kettlebell Breathing Technique

There are two kinds of breathing that kettlebells: Anatomical Breathing and Paradoxical Breathing. If you are engaged in short intense, heavy, high-intensity training, you must utilize the paradoxical breathing. The set which lasts for longer and has a lower weight should be supported through anatomical breathing.

Paradoxical Breathing

In this form of breathing you breathe in during the eccentric portion of the exercise and exhale when you reach the concentric part. For example, in squats, you take a breath on the way down and exhale while going up.

Anatomical Breathing

Anatomical breathing is a reverse of the paradoxical breathing. You breathe in during the concentric portion of the motion and exhale in the eccentric portion. This breathing style is perfect for endurance training.

Chapter 7: Workout Routine

Benefits of switching up the workout

In recent times it was observed that monotony in your fitness routine can be beneficial to your health, but it may not produce the desired result. Because it is essential to mix up the workouts frequently to ensure the maximum level of fitness. Alongside this variety of fitnessroutine, the routine can activate different muscles, both small and gigs. Kettlebell training is the most comprehensive training session that lasts a lifetime mixing cardio and strength aspects, but it is important to test different exercises with kettlebells to get additional advantages. Furthermore, it helps keep from becoming bored by avoiding repetition of the same routine each day and encourages you to learn more methods and exercises. Apart from that it also has the following benefits:

Muscles Development: If one follows the same routine of exercise each day, it could result in workouts becoming less effective over time. This can be due to two factors; firstly the muscles engaged in daily activity are exhausted, which can decrease the gains. Additionally, the muscles that aren't being utilized are not being used which could not give the desired results. It is therefore crucial to modify the exercise routine to increase the energy of your body, especially for those who are regular exercise. Professional athletes focus on specific workouts that build muscles that are specifically designed for their specific sport. A variety of exercises will help you build an athletic heart, muscular legs, as well as a strong upper body. This is achieved by setting a schedule for your workouts such as your schedule for the month could include aerobic and weight lifting exercises. This can help build strength, flexibility and increase the endurance of the entire body at the same time.

Weight Loss: People who want to shed weight usually stop it because they do the same routine each day that makes their body habituated to it. This is why even after performing the same workouts and making the same effort however, they fail to lose weight. In order to solve this problem it is recommended that people be encouraged to challenge their body with new workouts. This will force the body to adapt to new movements and also to start from a place of total inexperience by giving the body the chance to do something completely new in order to adapt. Although it will require greater effort, it can help burn more calories throughout the workout. Additionally when you are trying to shed weight it is essential to eat a balanced diet and avoid foods that can cause weight gain.

To prevent injuries: It has been discovered that repeated exercises could increase the likelihood of causing injuries including strain injury. This is due to the excessive use of muscles, which makes them tired to function effectively. To avoid this, it's essential to incorporate a variety of exercises in order to give an opportunity to work new ligaments and muscle groups. However the muscles that have been overused get time to heal and recover. In the event injuries, diversifying your exercises can allow you to do another sport that doesn't stress the same area of the body. This can help keep you in good shape and healing while healing. For instance bodybuilders split their workouts into distinct muscle groups, which allows various joints, muscles, and ligaments to relax while taking care not to put stress on their bodies when they exercise. If people persist in doing the same workout even after an injury, it could result in a more serious problem which could require months to heal.

To prevent boredom, there are many chances that someone will get bored if they do the same routine throughout the exercise and be unable to keep up with it. Since repetitive workouts can stress your body, but they don't aid in achieving the desired results. Furthermore that without the resistance, muscle exercise and a higher heart rate, your workout will not be effective. To achieve this it is crucial to keep motivation in the gym by trying new exercises within the training routine and always exploring new techniques. For instance, someone who likes weightlifting can only enroll in a Zumba class or other anaerobic workouts. This can help learn more about and identify what exercises are more appropriate for your body. Additionally, when a person begins a new exercise routine, it can help establish a new method as they learn how to improve and learn new techniques. This can eventually motivate those who are not able to complete the exercise and will keep their spirits up.

Healthy Brain: Engaging in exercises on a regular basis help to enhance the brain's performance by preventing the loss of memory in individuals. Additionally, challenging and trying new exercises daily aids the brain in developing new abilities and help keep neurons working effectively. It is crucial to choose the right workout to avoid injuries or overtraining. Studies show that those who don't have an unhealthy lifestyle and lead active lives have lower risks of developing high cholesterol, diabetes hypertension, stroke and diabetes.

Socializing: There's an opportunity to meet new people when one decides to try different workouts to working out. This will also assist in helping remain active, dedicated to a routine of exercise by identifying individuals who share your interests and who have the same objectives. It could also inspire you to take on new workouts together with other people.

Better Physique A person who is able to engage in a variety of activities in their workout routine are able to build fitness and are physically fit. Exercise helps strengthen muscles and enhance the general performance of the body. It is advised to experiment with new exercises over time based on the abilities of the person.

How to Change Your Workout Routine

As we have discussed, it is important to modify your routine of exercise by adding new exercises as time goes by. To be sure that there is no negative impact on your body, it's important to conduct a thorough research or speak with a professional before choosing a new exercise. Furthermore it is recommended to test something new starting at a an elementary level, for example for instance, if a person is spending thirty minutes riding a stationary bicycle, then he could intensify the exercise by increasing the speed or doing 10 of the 30 minutes on the treadmill.

Furthermore, there are many indications that suggest that one should alter their exercise routine. These typically include that an individual, despite maintaining an appropriate diet, is unable to detect any physical changes in their body. This suggests that there's an opportunity to experiment with different exercises that could prove beneficial to the body. Furthermore the fact that if a person doesn't feel hungry following the workout, it is important to alter the workouts. During exercise the body is working to repair the muscle fibers that are destroyed during exercise. It requires protein and nutrients to create a new protein strands. This is the reason that people feel hungry after an exercise session. When the workouts are easy, there aren't any muscles to repair and the body doesn't require any additional food.

Chapter 8: Literature Review

It is easy to gauge the efficacy of kettlebells through the increasing use in gyms around the world , and the positive effects have been made to the lives of a lot of people. People who train using kettlebells have discovered their power and strength to grow while enjoying more enjoyment due to the speciality of training with kettlebells.

What does the research on kettlebells reveal? Due to the growing popularity of kettlebells for training, kettlebells are now the subject of an extensive amount of scientific and academic research. In this section, we'll shift the focus from anecdotal to the academic, and examine what the studies are saying. All the sources will be listed in the following paragraphs.

Enhances explosive and maximal strength

One of the greatest benefits to training with kettlebells is that it results in an increase in strength and power at the same time. It is possible to define strength as the capacity of lifting or carrying a substantial amount of weight. In contrast, power refers to the capacity to move weight quickly. Kettlebell training can increase total strength and the ability to quickly move an object.

According to research, a course of training with swings increased the maximum strength by nearly 10 percent over the course of six weeks. It also increased capacity for cardiovascular exercise and jump power. The study was conducted by testing healthy men prior to and after 6 weeks of the kettlebell swing and six weeks on an squat jump program. The healthy males who completed an exercise that was biweekly for 12 minutes for six weeks demonstrated an increase in their maximum force and power which suggests an improvement the cardiovascular strength.

The full body motion of the kettlebell swing implies you can build strength, and explosive leaping power can be developed simultaneously.

Two additional studies found that kettlebell exercise increases power and strength. One study was focused on the young population while the other focused on strength overall compared to barbell exercises. The last study showed an increase in the clean and jerk movements when using kettlebells and the transfer of strength and power to bodyweight and traditional training.

A less expensive alternative to traditional weight lifting.

It's not necessary to blow your budget and transform your backyard or garage into a fitness center in order to reap the advantages of exercise. Kettlebells have been proven to be an effective substitute for bars and other machines.

A specific research study published by the Journal of Strength and Conditioning Research has proven that kettlebells work as an alternative to traditional methods for weightlifting particularly when you consider the size, portability, and their relatively low cost when compared to barbells weight plates as well as benches, squat racks and squat racks. A properly-planned training program using kettlebells could result in the same improvements in power, strength and endurance, but at lower costs and less space requirements. The research shows that kettlebell training can have the same results as other traditional methods of training for strength.

Improved cardiovascular fitness

Kettlebells are a good method to boost your metabolic rate, VO2 max (the ability of your body to carry oxygen A higher vo2 max typically means a greater amount in endurance) and to burn calories.

One study revealed that a simple regimen of kettlebell movements produced the identical "metabolic cost" similar to walking fast along an inclined treadmill. This means that a session that consists of, as in the case in the research, alternate with 10 swings as well as 10 deadlifts with kettlebells trained the cardiovascular system at the same level as treadmill walking. This was done at a lower intensity and a greater perceived level of effort, and also increased heart rate.

Benefits for the mind

Another study showed the use of kettlebells as a part of a shift to an active lifestyle was responsible an impact on mental health overall benefits. In the study, kettlebell exercise "increased overall happiness, well-being as well as self-reported strength, which are important psychological factors that could be considered as an alternative to the more conventional approaches to fitness".

I believe that the novelty and creativity of kettlebells training provides this psychological advantage. Training with kettlebells is enjoyable and can feel like a tough workout once it's completed. It is possible that you have had similar experiences during your own training in which knowing that you have got through a challenging exercise can provide a huge mental energy boost. Exercise that is effective also aids in the release of chemical substances that reduce stress and create positive mental health.

Tabata training

The most popular form of exercise is Tabata Training, and it has been proven in numerous study studies as an an extremely efficient in burning calories and boost your metabolism.

The Tabata protocol is named for Tabata, Dr. Izumi Tabata and was created in the 90's as an effective training method for speed skaters and cyclists. The protocol has since gained popularity and is being implemented to a variety of different disciplines. One of them can be Cross Fit, and many Cross Fit gyms use the Tabata method in their exercises.

What is the problem? The Tabata protocol repeats intervals of high intensity. The repeat is constructed around eight cycles of 20 seconds each on 10-second intervals. If you've been familiar with sprint-interval training (SIC) It has its roots in the Tabata protocol.

The study examined the Tabata Protocol kettlebell workout with the sprint-interval (SIC) training session on stationary bicycles. The SIC workout consisted of 30 second, full-intensity sprints followed by a 4 minute break. The Tabata kettlebell exercise was designed using the 20/10 sequence. It included sumo squats, swings, press and clean to sumo deadlifts.

The study concluded that Tabata type of workout that involves kettlebell movements resulted in a increased V2max (your body's ability to generate oxygen and use it to be better able to sustain prolonged, sustained effort) as well as calorie burning and positive metabolic and cardiovascular changes.

Talk about value for your buck. By incorporating this four minute workout into your workout routine, you will be able to boost your metabolism and increase mitochondria power.

Chapter 9: Kettlebell Training

Kettlebells are a type of strength-training equipment that have been praised for some time. The kettlebells consist of iron ball that vary between 5 and 100 pounds. Kettlebells were first introduced in Russia and are beginning to become popular throughout the USA.

Kettlebells provide a unique type of exercise because it targets nearly every muscle within the body. It is also used to improve balance, endurance and agility as well as resistance cardio training.

The principle of kettlebell training is holding the weight with just one or both hands and go through a sequence of motions such as swings, pulling motions or presses. Certain exercises require you move the weight around while you move. This lets you work your core muscles more.

The difference between dumbbells and dumbbells

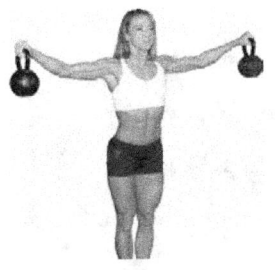

Many people think of kettlebells as dumbbells. The primary difference between kettlebells and dumbbells is the design. The handle of kettlebells is different from the way it affects the body.

If you are using dumbbells, the weight is placed on your hands, but when kettlebells are used the weight is transferred out of the hand, which means it is able to alter based on the movement you make. The majority of kettlebell exercises are focused on centrifugal force, which transfers the weight evenly to muscles. These kinds of movements are akin to the real-world exercises. They are excellent to build muscles through controlled movements, while kettlebells can be utilized for full body exercises using fluid exercises.

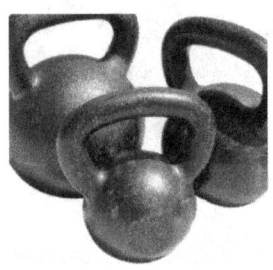

Benefits of kettlebell exercise

It's a mix of fitness and cardio. Kettlebell training is like running, but with a heavier burden.

• Burns additional fat. Kettlebells exercise is a combination of explosive movements which make use of muscles and increase the metabolic capacity that the body.

Exercises with kettlebells can increase your coordination and agility.

It helps strengthen alignment muscles , which result in better posture.

It's efficient and time-saving. Kettlebell exercises let you exercise multiple parts in your own body.

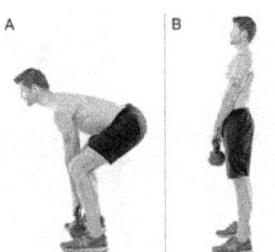

Aid you in becoming more effective in other forms of exercise.

Increases endurance and stamina.

It's a good way to keep injuries at bay. Kettlebell can help you with eccentric deceleration, which helps increase the strength of the body.

- Simplicity. The equipment is simple to use and the majority of exercises are simple.

- Time efficient. Individuals who do not have time to get to the gym may opt to engage in a short amount of kettlebell exercises for a total fitness routine.

- Calorie burning capabilities. On average, individuals can burn up to 1,200 calories when they do kettlebell exercises.

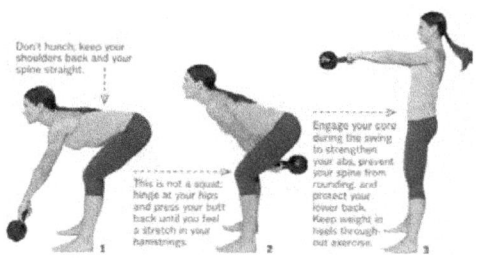

Kettlebell security

Like any other workout individuals must be aware of the appropriate precautions when using kettlebells. Kettlebells requires coordination, strength, and practice. It is essential to begin your exercise slowly and increase the intensity as you advance. Beware of lifting kettlebells that are heavy for those who are just beginning because it could cause numerous injuries.

Basic kettlebell exercises

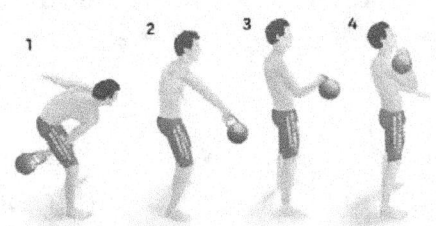

Dead lift

A lot of kettlebell exercises rely on dead lift exercises. Dead lifts are great to relax hip reflectors, as well as building the quad muscle. It's a good idea to master this fundamental move as it is the base of all other movements.

Keep your feet about an inch apart. Move your toes a little towards the outside. Make sure you position yourself as if would like to sit in the chair. Maintain your heels down. Take the kettlebell in both hands. Make sure you maintain your hands straight. The kettlebell should be lifted to the point that your legs remain straight. Don't extend your arms, and don't apply pressure to your back. Your body should be in an upright line when standing. The kettlebell should be lowered and you can repeat the exercise.

Swing

Two-arm swings are always utilized for kettlebell training. It is considered to be an exercise for the whole body and can be utilized to improve the power of dead lifts as well as squats.

Keep your feet separated. Put the weight in between the heels of your feet. Lower your body, and grasp the kettlebell's handle using both hands. The arms must be in a straight line and the shoulders still. Your weight should be on your heels, not on your toes.

Your hips should be pushed towards the kettlebell, then swing it forward. Let the kettlebell move back towards your butt. Once the kettlebell is under your butt, push your hips forward , then move the kettlebell until it gets to your chest. Then let your arms go back and forth until the kettlebell is behind you. Keep your head elevated and you're back in a straight line.

Clean and press

Cleaning and pressing is an essential kettlebell movement that requires full body movements. Begin by straddling your kettlebell. Maintain your feet wide apart. Squat, and hold the handle using one hand by using the grip with an overhand. Your shoulder should be placed over the kettlebell and keep your spine straight.

1. Take the kettlebell off of the floor and then push your hips upwards.

2. When the kettlebell has landed above the ground, you can pull it up over your shoulders and let your elbow be bent to the side.

3. After the kettlebell has been placed on your chest, turn your elbow in front of the kettlebell.

4. You can grab the kettlebell by using the outside of your arms. Keep your wrist straight , and bend your knees. It is also known rack position.

5. Lift the kettlebell from your arm, and then secure it above your head.

6. Lower the kettlebell, then return in the position of rack. Lower the kettlebell until it is on the ground, and repeat the exercise.

Get ready

Getup is regarded among the most simple but challenging kettlebell exercises. It involves the entire body and improves stabilization and stability. It is advised to use a kettlebell that is lighter for the getup novices.

1. Relax and place the kettlebell by your side. Keep the kettlebell in your right hand , and then extend the kettlebell to the level of your chest.

2. Flex your left leg to ensure you have your foot close to your butt. Maintain the left leg in a straight position, and move your left arm to the side. Arms on the right should extend fully over your head. Push your chest out.

3. Lift your right shoulder upwards and utilize your left elbow to provide

assistance. Place the kettlebell over your head.

4. Transfer from left elbow towards the right. Make sure your right arm is fully extended.

5. Lift your hips up and tighten your glutes.

6. Move your left leg in front of you until you have your knee on the ground. This is also known as the lunge posture. Make sure you stand up and hold the arms in a straight line.

Chapter 10: Nutrition

It's not a good idea to say the notion that diet is one-size for all type of exercise. Certain rules should be adhered to in order to guarantee your body's change. It is important to ensure that you are taking in enough protein without putting too much calories. Macronutrients are crucial. For a healthy and fit body, your body needs the proper nutrients in the proper quantities. Many people go down the wrong path when they make the decision to die and do so by cutting down on the caloric intake. This means reducing the amount of carbs. This is true in the case of sweets, sugar and bread. If the body is subjected to radical changes in diet, it adjusts to chemical processes and seeks to protect the stores of glucose.

Carbohydrates are the primary source of energy , which fuels the muscle's performance. Carbohydrates break down our bodies into small components that can be utilized by the body. They are stored in the form of glycogen within muscles liver and fat, and can be used when needed. This is why extreme changes that are sudden and drastic could be detrimental since when the body detects an increase in the amount of glycogen it will adjust to protect the existing. In other words, metabolism slows in order to conserve energy. In times of extreme deficiency in carbohydrates, when glycogen stores have been depleted, the body is able to metabolize the protein it produces to supply energy. This results in the loss of skin hairs on the muscles and bones, making the body appear as being hungry.

Apart from providing the energy for growth and cellular function, carbohydrates also play these functions in the body

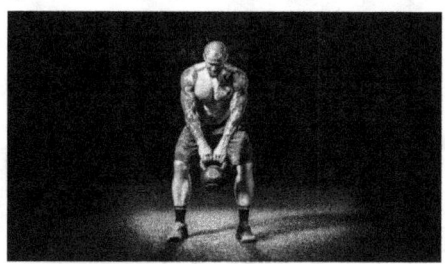

Regulate blood sugar levels

Aids in the absorption of calcium

Help probiotics get nutrients from the colon

Helps in controlling cholesterol and blood pressure levels.

The CNS is powered by fuel and the brain

When it comes to maintaining a healthy diet, choosing protein, vitamins and minerals that come from natural sources and at the all times avoiding processed foods is the most crucial measure to ensure the health of your.

A proper diet includes the following elements:

Proteins from lean fish meats and nuts

Fruits and vegetables

When it comes to grains and other carbs like barley corn meal, beans and

Dairy, including milk cheese and yogurt

Oils and healthy fats

There are a few refined grains like potatoes, white rice

Very little of other things such as alcohol and salt sugar.

There is no one ideal diet program that can meet the requirements of each person and when you are planning your diet, the common sense and a little information about ingredients and nutrition is essential. Be sure to take into consideration the below

Be aware of the portion sizes. You should eat less and not eat more.

Pick from a range of foods that can provide you with the nutrition you require

In each meal, the type of carbs consumed should be carefully selected

Always select foods that are high-quality. More natural, less processed.

Always have breakfast and healthy snacks, between midmorning and in the afternoon.

Make sure you add a small amount of protein that is lean.

Avoid caffeine and drink only green tea

Never underestimate the importance of keep well hydrated. Make sure you drink plenty of water.

Mix in spices and herbs to aid in digestion

When exercising, it's crucial to stay well-hydrated in order to replenish the sweat-loss fluids. The intensity of workouts can result in massive water demands that can be as high as 2-3 gallons water each day. Water is essential to perform the following functions.

The fluid component of blood, which transports oxygen as well as other nutrients.

Eliminates the cellular waste products and toxins from the body in a solution

Aids in the thermoregulation process.

Helps improve digestion

Chapter 11: Many benefits of Kettlebell Training

There are many exercise tools and equipment on the market. They're all extremely efficient and offer each with its own advantages. I'll never inform anyone that one piece or piece of exercise equipment is not suitable for you. Particularly if you have experienced positive results. I'll recommend that a specific kind of tool is more efficient and useful in the event that it has all the features of several tools at once. For instance, a Swiss knives is definitely more effective than a normal pocket knife. Whatever your fitness objectives may be, the kettlebell could aid you in reaching them. The most important thing that we have discussed in the chapter 2 is to make sure you choose the kettlebell that is most suitable for your needs.

Kettlebell exercises are the benefits of cardiovascular training and strength training. These are two primary areas that lead to muscle development as well as fat reduction and weight loss as well as general well-being. Due to the intense nature of the exercises and the wide range of body parts targeted by each one, you'll notice an extreme burn of fat and muscle building within a matter of minutes. I have noticed this in a significant way and have been training since you can recall.

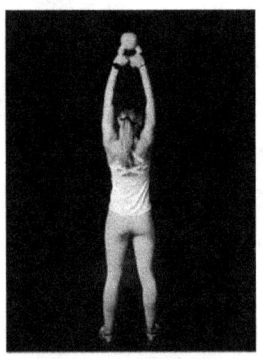

If this story isn't appealing enough to you, think about a few other options. An ex-top fighter of K1, Bob Sapp, has been a big fan of kettlebells to increase his cardio through his training. Former UFC Welterweight champion BJ Penn is a kettlebell trainer to boost his strength and endurance. Bob Sapp and BJ Penn both Bob Sapp and BJ Penn have experienced huge success against top fighters from their respective clubs. Hollywood actor Ed O'Neil, who is an avid fan of Brazilian Jiu-Jitsu, is an avid fan of kettlebells training. It is receiving increasingly praised by fitness enthusiasts all over the world and is gaining momentum more than ever before.

This could be one of the main reasons why people consider it to be an fad. When celebrities start to jump on different trends, it's difficult to determine whether they're serious or just looking to gain publicity. As I said before kettlebells have been in use for centuries, but only began to gain international attention in the decade of 2000. It's not a trend since a lot of practitioners across the globe sing about its benefits. That includes me. The kettlebell has been a godsend for me, far above what I was experiencing during my most sporting days. This equipment can help you out too.

CARDIOVASCULAR and STRENGTH Training

There are a lot of exercises that offer incredible cardio and strength training. But, few of them combine these two together. The most common kettlebell routines, such as cleans, swings, snatches and jerks work the entire body as one unit. In essence, you work on a variety of body and muscle parts in just a few minutes, and the exercises are challenging. You'll feel them in an intense way and likely put in the most effort you previously.

Exercises with kettlebells that are ballistic such as high rep snatches make sprinting appear like a stroll on the beach. However, it isn't like that. The rep snatches will also work more muscles than sprinting and significantly improve strength in the shoulders, lower back and hips. Through the many high-intensity workouts that can be done using a kettlebell muscle will be challenged unlike anything else.

Recent studies have revealed that swings can produce as much as 20 calories in a minute. This is 400 calories for a 20 minute workout if performed correctly. It's an extremely high rate of burning calories. In addition, because of the intensity, you'll experience the afterburn. That means that you're producing calories at an fast level even after the workout is finished. You'd have be running for a longer duration with at least a 6 minute mile speed to even get close to these numbers.

Kettlebell training is more attractive for males than other options like spin classes or step aerobics. Men are generally concerned about their fitness and feel as if they're fools when they practice them. This makes them unable to achieve the fitness level they want and need. I'm not knocking these workouts. I believe they're fantastic. This is just an assertion of real-world situation here. Men feel more confident exercising with kettlebells that have ballistic design over something similar to Zumba. You can take your kettlebell workouts to the next level by mixing them up with other exercises like jogging or jump roping.

The use of kettlebells can improve the strength of our functional muscles as well. It is due to the fact that it mimics the movements of our muscles and functions in their natural condition. Our muscles don't work independently. They collaborate with each other to prevent over-strain on the muscles, prevent injuries, perform better and strengthen. For instance the muscles in our legs do not work on their own while walking. The effort is spread across the entire body, and everything is working efficiently. Kettlebell training is based on the same principle. If we can learn to utilize our muscles with a variety of techniques for training, this can carry into the practicality of our daily lives. By using the correct methods for functional training you can lower the chance of injury in your daily lives and also increase your agility, strength as well as flexibility and balance.

Kettlebells will also improve the strength of your core as well as stability. Because many kettlebell exercises are ballistic They focus on rapid movements, maximizing acceleration and decreasing deceleration. Abdominal muscles are stimulated heavily through these movements because of their intensities and the core contracting. Make sure you align your core contractions using appropriate breathing because of the intensity. Your core strength improve dramatically and even more than when you do targeted exercises such as leg raises or crunches. Additionally, kettlebell exercises place less stress to your spine and do not require you to lie on the floor like crunches require. Of course, there are some specific exercises for crunches which we'll discuss.

The kettlebell exercises your core in different directions since they're multiplanar. The unilateral exercises also provide significant strength and stability to your core. You'll see a significant increase in the strength of your core after only a handful of exercises. Once you are able to perform various exercises at any level you'll be able to be able to understand the meaning of core engagement.

Many athletes train using the kettlebell due to this reason. They require a high level of core strength to get through their competition and change direction at a moment's notice and handle massive load from either direction. Training using kettlebells can give a person the strength and endurance to take on the pressures of these kinds. Mike Tyson was one of the most fierce heavyweight boxers ever recorded. Tyson would take down his foes and then slam them over the head at a glance.

The most interesting part is that Tyson wasn't a massive man. In any case, not in comparison to the heavier giants that are out there. So how was he able to push others around the ring without having to be pushed and back? Due to his incredible fundamental strength. He was a rock solid player in this area. This allowed him to move forward, side-to-side and make any last-minute adjustments if necessary. He was able to take the impact of punches hitting his body due to this reason. If the kettlebell could give athletes of professional grade the fundamental strength they require think about what it could provide for your daily needs. Strength is vital to becoming an athlete of the highest caliber.

One aspect of strength-training that is often overlooked is grip strength. It's kind of funny because one of the most common ways two individuals test their strength is when shaking their hands. It is likely the hand shake is an typical issue in any exercise routine. But, a bad grip will cause you to suffer big disadvantages when doing a range of exercises. A solid grip can allow you to lift heavier weights. Additionally, the more solid you grip the bigger as well as stronger the forearms be. The kettlebell has greatly increased grip strength of a lot of people who have tried it.

There are two elements that are at work here. In the first place, the handle is bigger than a standard dumbbell, which means that your grip will be more strained. Additionally, the nature of kettlebell workouts will place greater stress than normal on your forearms and hands which will result in more involvement of muscles that are located in the region. For instance the swing demands you to keep the kettlebell in your hand for a prolonged time frame, and you must contend with a constantly shifting the center of gravity. All of this leads to a stronger grip. After a while of training with a kettlebell to the top and rub your pals hands. They'll be awestruck. Don't grip too hard. You don't want to cause harm them.

The kettlebell will greatly increase your endurance and strength. You will not only be more comfortable in your exercise routines as well as in your day-to-day life. You'll be able to have more energy for running your the errands. The stairs will not seem to be as intimidating. Whatever you like to do you, it will be much easier to enjoy them since you'll have more energy. You'll not be as exhausted at work, which means that you are more productive. The kettlebell workout will improve your general health and well-being as an entire.

Balance and Power

If you're running on a treadmill, or using the majority of other machines, you are operating along a specific path. There aren't many directions that you can run in on the treadmill. Even if you're inventive, you're very limited in the number of muscles you are able to engage. With a kettlebell, you are able to expand your moves. To achieve this, you have to increase the stabilizing muscle every time. If you combine this increase in strength of the stabilizer muscles along with the strength of the core we talked about earlier the balance you have will become incredible. This is basically the process of building stability through instability.

Kettlebell training can help your balance as it teaches you to be able to cope with the constant shift in your centre of gravity. By adjusting the postures and stances you adopt throughout your workout the center of gravity for the kettlebell lies at least 6-8 inches in front of the grip. This means you have to contend with an force that tests your balance, something you'll encounter frequently in the daily activities you engage in.

As an offshoot of balance kettlebells are great to improve posture. Many exercises are designed to target all of the backside. This encompasses your middle, upper, and lower back, as well as your hamstrings, glutes, and traps. All the muscles within these areas will grow very strong and will lead to an improved posture. The strengthening of your core muscles in the neck muscles, shoulders and hips will help you achieve this too.

We have previously discussed strength and kettlebell exercise can significantly increase your endurance strength across all parts of your body. The kettlebell can also increase the power output of your body. This is more than strength. It refers to the ability to generate forces over a prolonged time. Power is an additional element of it because it is related more to the adversity of the movements concerned. Power is the body's capacity to produce the maximum amount of force in the quickest time feasible. Kettlebell training helps in this process by forcing you to perform rapid and powerful movements repeatedly and over. The power of your movements is the main factor in the majority of athletic competitions.

In terms of power In terms of power, let's think about our good friend Mike Tyson again. There's no doubt that Mike is a powerful man. If you pit him against a competitor from a competition , and they engage in an obstacle course The strongman is likely to take the victory. He'll be able produce more force in longer periods of time. If the two were to compete in a fight, Mike Tyson would probably triumph because he is able to produce an increased force in a shorter time which means he has greater explosiveness. In essence, the strongman is more powerful, however Tyson is more strong.

DON'T FEEL PAIN!

The main benefit of kettlebell exercise is the dramatic reduction in pain across the body. A lot of people suffer from lower back pain because of the weak glute muscles that comprise the buttocks region. They are the biggest muscles in the body , and they are the primary reason for most movements. If they are weak, they are unable to take on the load that they need to which means that a large portion of the burden falls on their lower back muscles. The muscles of the lower back aren't designed to support the same load as glutes do. In time the lower back will begin suffering from strain and pain can become a major issue. This could result in major injuries later on that can become crippling. When we build the glute muscles by doing regular kettlebell exercises and exercises, they are given the ability to begin carrying their own weight. This will greatly reduce the burden on the back, and will effectively decrease lower back pain.

A major pain resulting from arthritis is also preventable if kettlebell exercises can improve and keep joint health in good shape. Different exercises require deliberate control of movements which helps strengthen your muscles which support joints. Furthermore the increased elasticity in the tendons and ligaments can improve mobility and to prevent serious injuries such as strains, sprains and tears. You'll become more durable overall.

CONVENIENCE, AND OTHER Benefits

We've discussed many advantages in the kettlebell. One of the best advantages of them is the ease of use. It is possible to exercise frequently and vigorously without needing to go to an exercise facility. If it's pouring, snowing or hailing, you'll have this equipment available. You just need to walk into in your room, where else you might put it in, then begin your workout with a variety of exercises. In just 20 minutes of intense training, you'll be sweaty and soaked and will feel a feeling of satisfaction having have completed a fantastic exercise.

If you don't be at home and work out then you don't need to. The kettlebell is lightweight and can be taken across a range of places. If you are feeling that you require a breath of fresh air, you can take the kettlebell to the local park and practice some basic moves there. You can also have one at work to perform some repetitions in your breaks. Be sure not to sweat excessively while in the workplace. It's not the best image for a workplace. If you enjoy exercising at the gym, there's a good chance they'll include kettlebells in the gym too.

The most important thing is the fact that you can use this multi-functional device almost everywhere. It's very easy to use and can provide an excellent exercise at the touch of an eye. There is no other equipment needed. You may utilize other equipments if you prefer. Like we said before that there are a variety of exercises that complement the kettlebell, however, there are few of them can be used to replace it. Another aspect of kettlebell exercises that I haven't highlighted yet is that they're very enjoyable to perform. It is likely that you won't miss doing any other activity. I'll say it is wonderful not having to think about kettlebells at home and can be kept in a closet or in a corner opposed to a treadmill or an ellipticalthat takes the entire living space.

There are numerous additional benefits that kettlebells provide. The exercises can be utilized to help you recover from an active workout. Recovering properly is crucial for active people or athletes all over the world. It is true that lying on the couch and eating unhealthy food isn't an effective recovery method. You'll be with a lower energy level and be in worse shape as you were. If you decide to jump back into your exercise routine it is like getting back to square one. The most important thing is to keep the level of fitness. This can be accomplished by doing some simple exercises that bring blood to the muscle groups that have been working.

This can help speed the recovery process significantly and help keep you fit between intense exercises.

A way to utilize kettlebells effectively to recover is to follow the training regimens that are taught by Jeff Martone, who is the Physical Training and Combative Coordinator of the Direct Action Resource Center. Jeff. Martone knows a lot about training. Through his numerous videos, he covers numerous kettlebell drills in which you move the kettlebell from one hand to another hands in the air in mid-air. Apart from ensuring blood flow in muscles, these exercises enhance the hand-eye control, strength of grip as well as the ability to take in shock. The exercises test your brain, meaning that not only will your physically exhausted, but also mentally exhausted as well.

We've already mentioned it previously, but we will remind you that kettlebell exercises are a great way to save time. If you had the option of choosing between a workout lasting 20 minutes or 60 minutes and both burn the same amount of calories. Which would you prefer? When it comes to workouts, quality is much more than the quantity. If you've been to the gym a number of time, you've likely noticed the differing levels of exertion put into by different people. A person is working hard and working to their limits and another person is just performing the routine. The person who is more focused will see substantially better results, regardless of regardless of how long the other spends. To achieve great results it is essential to be more than present. You must be completely involved.

When the kettlebell is utilized correctly, you'll achieve astonishing results. You'll burn the exact amount of calories in just 20 minutes, as you would after an hour of cycling or running. Also, consider how much you push yourself during these workouts. Imagine picking up a kettlebell during the morning, in the afternoon, or evening, and then doing the most intense exercises for 20 minutes, and feeling great afterward. You didn't even have to leave your home to fix your hair, or appear attractive at all. It was just a matter of getting started, and you finished before you realized you could. It's not a fantasy and a reality. 20 minutes per day, for at the very least several days in a week is certainly doable no matter what your schedule is. The aspect that you don't need to leave your house is a plus. This "I don't have the time" excuse is not a valid one in this case. Time is available; all you need is to make use of it.

The kettlebell is an incredible product. My sole regret is not having discovered it earlier in my the course of my life. With all the wonderful benefits, it's difficult to ignore it as an investment worth it. If you are concerned about the price consider comparing it to the cost of a gym membership per month or the different exercise equipment needed to take care of all the areas of your body. Additionally, think about other expenses you can eliminate or cut down on that help you pay for. I'm not a financial planner, and I'm not planning to get too deep into this. A thing to consider is that, once you've got an excellent kettlebell or two it will last quite a long time. The earlier you get one the more effective. Get it and take possession of it.

Chapter 12: Intermediate Kettlebell Exercises

This chapter I'll take your upper core, lower, and upper kettlebell exercises to the next stage by offering intermediate exercises.

Before performing any of the exercises in Chapter 2, you should practice the exercises using a kettlebell. Be aware of the way your body moves throughout the exercise , and be aware of any weak points or imbalances that may arise. Make sure you are in good shape without adding weight before bringing your kettlebell to the gym. Form is essential in getting the most of your workout and avoiding injuries.

Tips: It's always an excellent idea to think about taking a few sessions with a kettlebell coach to help you improve your technique. Professionals can observe your movements in an objective way from different angles and offer direction to ensure you're doing each move when you exercise correctly.

Important note: Many of the exercises during the workouts require placing the kettlebell in a racked, stacked position. Refer to the description and illustration at the end of chapter 5 for those who are new to the sport.

Squats and Lunges If you're having issues with your knees and have difficulty doing lunges or squats, just take it as far as you are able to comfortably. As you gain strength, you may try sliding lower. If you're not able to perform an entire squat or lunge, continue to perform the exercise at a safe range for the joints.

When to increase the weight or repetitions When to increase reps or weight: Refer the chapter for tips for when you should raise the weight of your kettlebell or repetitions or sets.

Intermediate Upper BODY KETTLEBELL TRAINING

Intermediate Upper BODY KETTLEBELL Workout

SETS FOR EXERCISE REPS

Shoulder salutation 8-10 3 5

Clean and press 8 - 10. 3 5

Overhead squat 8 - 10 3 - 5

Burpee push up to 8-10 3 5

Single-handed deadlift 8-10 3 - 5

Rest time between sets: 30 seconds to 2 minutes. Reduce the time between sets as you advance and become stronger.

SHOULDER SALUTATION

Muscles targeted: Shoulders back and core, quads the hamstrings

Make sure your knees are bent and your body hinged upwards from your hips at a 45-degree angle with respect to the ground.

Hold your kettlebell either side of your body and then hold it up in front of you by extending your arms to the shoulder height. The arms must be parallel to the floor.

Then bend your knees to semi-squat and then increase your arms until they're in the exact 45 degree angle to your torso.

Maintain your spine straight throughout the exercise.

Return to your starting position with your knees bent slightly and your arms extended to the ground.

CLEAN and ROSE

Muscles to be targeted: Shoulders back quads, core, glutes, hamstrings, and hamstrings.

Place your feet shoulder width apart, with your kettlebell with the racked posture. This is the exact position in which you'll finish the repetitions in.

Then extend your elbow and then swing the kettlebell downwards. While it's swinging downward make sure you bend your knees to move your torso forward with your hips. Allow your kettlebell to move through your legs.

When your kettlebell begins to swing forward once more then straighten your legs and bring your torso to a standing position. When you are straightening, move your hips forward. The force generated by your hip thrust can boost the momentum of your kettlebell's upward movement.

When your kettlebell is swinging upwards Bend your elbow and bring it back to the racked posture.

From the inverted position, raise your arms straight overhead and do a press. Make sure the arm remains straight and aligned with your elbow, wrist, and shoulder aligned with one another.

Return to the rack position.

Alternative: Clean and Push Press

Make sure you clean it up and do the extra bit by performing an incline half. Complete your clean to make your kettlebell move into the rack position. Before performing the press, you should do an squat half. When you are able to push up out of the half-squat position to an upright position, you can make use of the momentum to raise your arms into the press.

SQUAT OVERHEAD

Muscles to be targeted: shoulders, glutes, core and quads. Hamstrings, glutes, glutes

Place your feet shoulder width apart, keeping the kettlebell to the rack position.

From the inverted position, move your arm straight overhead in order to press. Be sure that the arm remains straight and aligned with your elbow, wrist, and shoulder aligned with one another.

Bend your knees and pull your torso to the side from your hips for an Squat. Maintain your back straight.

Return to a standing posture.

BURPEE PULLL Up

The muscles targeted are: the shoulder, back, core glutes, hamstrings, glutes

You should be in a comfortable, neutral posture; feet shoulder width apart, and place your kettlebell in between your feet.

Bend your knees, and then hinge your torso to the side from the hips to complete the Squat.

Your hands should be wide enough to be shoulder-width apart on either end of the kettlebell.

Maintain your arms straight.

In a quick, fluid motion , jump your feet forward. Now you should be in a push-up or plank position.

Do one push-up.

Move your feet both forwards to get into an upright squatting position using your hands on either side of the kettlebell.

Grab the top of your kettlebell with both hands.

Stand up again and lift your kettlebell along with you.

Don't stop your kettlebell's kinetics. Bend your elbows and then bring the kettlebell towards your chest. Make sure your elbows are towards the side and parallel to the ground.

Lower your kettlebell down to the thigh height.

Sit down and put your kettlebell between your feet.

Variations:

Burpee Clean Replace your pull-up with a kettlebell clean changing the workout in the following manner:

Then, with both feet, jump forward to ensure that you're standing squatting position with your hands placed on the opposite sides of the kettlebell.

Grab the top of your kettlebell with one hand.

While you are straightening, thrust your hips inwards, the strength generated by the thrust of your hips can boost the momentum of the kettlebell's upward motion.

When your kettlebell is swinging upwards then bend your elbow to move it back into the racked position.

Move your elbow to the side and then swing your kettlebell in an upward angle. While it is going downward make sure you bend your knees inwards and pivot your torso to the side from your hips. Place your kettlebell back onto the floor between your feet.

Burpee Press: Swap the pull-up and do presses instead. Here's how to replace the movement:

Move your feet both forwards to get into an upright squatting position with your hands placed on the opposite side of the kettlebell.

Hold the top of the kettlebell with one hand.

While you are straightening, thrust your hips forward. The force generated by your hip thrust will boost the speed of the kettlebell's upward swing.

As the kettlebell moves upwards then bend your elbow to move it back into the racked position.

From the inverted position, raise your arms straight overhead in order to perform a push. Be sure that you are straight and aligned with your elbow, wrist and shoulder aligned with one another.

Return to the standing position.

Move your elbow to the side and swing your kettlebell into an upward arch. While it is swinging downward you should bend your knees, then move your torso forward with your hips. Place your kettlebell on the floor between your feet.

DEADLIFT SINGLE-HANDED

Muscles targeted: shoulders glutes, back, core and quads. Hamstrings, glutes,

Relax in a neutral position, with your feet shoulder-width apart, and your kettlebell in between your feet.

Bend your knees and bring your torso inwards from your hips. Keep your back straight.

Hold your kettlebell tightly by the handle using one hand.

Straighten yourself to a standing posture and then lift your kettlebell in front of your. The kettlebell should hang on your body at the level of your thighs.

Bend your knees and pivot your torso upwards from your hips until you can place the kettlebell back between your feet.

Keep the shoulders level and straight.

INTERMEDIATE CORE KETTLEBELL Workout

INTERMEDIATE CORE KETTLEBELL FOR WORKOUT

SETS FOR EXERCISE REPS

Sit up and press 8-10 3 - 5

Renegade row 8-10 per side, 3 5

Russian twist between 8 and 10 per side, 3 5

Mountain climbers 45-60 seconds between 3 and 5

Lateral bends 8-10 per side, 3 5

Rest time between sets: 30 seconds to 2 minutes. You can reduce the time between sets as you progress and you get stronger.

STAND UP, PRESS

The muscles targeted are: core, back and shoulders

Put your feet on the ground. Your legs must be straight towards you, or bent at your knee, which is similar to the posture used for regular sit-ups.

Hold your kettlebell by either side of the handle , then raise it towards your chest.

Lay back on the floor and hold your kettlebell on your chest.

Do a sit-up routine with your kettlebell held lightly in your chest. Do not push it toward the sky or allow it to fall to the floor.

When you are in a sitting posture then raise your kettlebell up for a double-hand press. Lower the kettlebell towards your chest.

Then lower yourself back to the floor.

It is important to activate your core muscles when performing the sit-up, do not strain your back muscles to keep from injury.

Alternative: Straight Arm Sit Up

Increase the intensity of this workout by holding your kettlebell with one hand and lying down to the ground. Lift your arm straight to lift your kettlebell up to the ceiling. Perform the sit-up while lifting your kettlebell up while keeping your arms towards the ceiling.

Renegade RROW

Muscles targeted: core glutes, glutes, shoulders toes, hamstrings, quads

To complete this exercise you'll require a kettlebell, as well as something that's approximately equal in height to the handle of your kettlebell. It is possible to use a wooden box, for instance.

Set your wooden box, or any other item of support and your kettlebell shoulder-width across on the floor.

Make sure you are in a push or plank up position by placing one hand placed on the support's top while the other hand is on the top of the kettlebell handle.

The kettlebell should be lifted above the floor, bent your elbow, then pulling it back toward the ceiling.

Reduce your kettlebell by extending your arm downwards toward the floor. Don't extend your arm, or place your kettlebell on the floor. Instead, hold it at a minimum of an inch from the floor.

RUSSIAN TWIST

The muscles targeted are: core, back shoulders, back

Place your feet on the floor and keep the knees bent.

Grab your kettlebell from the opposite side of the handle , then raise it towards your chest.

Lean backwards at a 45-degree angle.

Turn your body to the left and bring your kettlebell over your lap and to your left side.

Reduce your kettlebell so as to place it to your left, but keep it at a distance of about an inch above surface.

Your torso should be turned to the left, then bring the kettlebell onto your lap and to your right side.

The kettlebell should be lowered as if to lay it down on your right , but stop at a distance of about an inch above surface.

MOUNTAIN CLIMBERS

Muscles to be targeted: core, shoulders back, hamstrings glutes, quads

Take a plank or push up position, with the kettlebell positioned beneath your chest. You should keep your arms straightwith two hands together, gripping the handle tightly. The kettlebell should sit under your shoulders and your chest in a way that your wrist shoulder, and elbow are aligned with each other directly across the handle of the kettlebell.

You'll know the location on your kettlebell's axis is right when it doesn't wobble , or seem to threaten to collapse under your weight. If it is wobbling and are unable to maintain your position the kettlebell could be too far to the left. If the elbows are aligned and straight, your arms are locked in an even line between your shoulder and your wrist, and then the handle of your kettlebell.

After you've settled in a comfortable position, raise one knee toward your chest. Place all of your weight on the other leg as well as your arms.

Continue to extend your leg until it is back in position, repeating the opposite leg.

The goal of this exercise is to replicate the running motion of a high-knee while in a plank position. This will truly strengthen your muscles in your core.

LATERAL BEND

The muscles targeted are: the core, shoulders back, core

Place your feet at shoulder width, with your kettlebell firmly held in your left hand and lying on your side.

Place your weight on your left hip and then bend to the right as far as you are able to comfortably.

Keep your position to a number of one before readjusting your posture.

Intermediate LOWER BODY KETTLEBELL TRAINING

Intermediate LOWER BODY KETTLEBELL TRAINING

SETS FOR EXERCISE REPS

Single-handed kettlebell swing from 8 to 10 per side, 3 5

Racked squat , press 8-10 times per side. Each side should be 3 to 5

Press and lunge racked 8-10 - 10 each side from 3 to 5

Sumo square with back and front jumps between 8 and 10 3 5

Overhead double lunge 8 - 10 3 - 5

The rest period between sets is 30 seconds to 2 minutes. You can reduce the time between sets as you progress and you get stronger.

SINGLE-HANDED KETTLEBELL SWING

Muscles to be targeted: quads glutes, hamstrings Core and back

Place the feet spread shoulder width apart knees bent slightly and your torso swaying upwards from your hips. Maintain your back straight as your torso hinges forward.

Grab the top of your kettlebell with one hand.

Lift your kettlebell off of the ground , and let it slide back and forth across your legs.

Straighten your body to a standing point and then thrust your hips inwards. The thrust of your hips will provide an energy boost to your kettlebell swing.

The kettlebell should be thrown out to the side by arching it until it is at the height of your chest while keeping your elbow straight.

When your kettlebell begins to swing downwards once more Bend your knees, then pivot your body forward from your hips. Then allow the kettlebell to move between your legs.

RACKED SQUAT and Press

Muscles to be targeted: glutes quads, hamstrings back, core, glutes

Keep your feet shoulder-width apart with your kettlebell with the rack position.

Bend your knees and bring your torso inwards from your hips in order to do the lunge.

Remain in a standing position.

From the inverted position, raise your arms straight overhead in order to do a press. Make sure you are straight and aligned with your elbow, wrist, and shoulder aligned with one another.

The kettlebell should be lowered back into the rack position.

Variation Double Kettlebell Racked Squat and Press

If you own two kettlebells that have similar weight and weight, you can make the exercise more challenging by having two bells with one hand and in the racked position to increase the weight of resistance.

RACKED LUNGE, Press

Muscles to be targeted: glutes quads, hamstrings, shoulders back, core, glutes

Keep your feet shoulder-width apart keeping the kettlebell to the rack position.

Move into a lunge posture by either moving back into the reverse lunge or moving forward into a normal lunge.

When you are performing the lunge, you should extend your arm straight overhead in order to press. Be sure that your arms are straight and your elbow, wrist, and shoulder aligned with one another.

Remain in a standing position and return your kettlebell to its racked state in the same manner as you did.

While performing the lunge, the side on which you hold the kettlebell should be on the same side that you are holding it on as your forward-facing knee.

Tips: If doing the lunge and press simultaneously is too difficult, do the lunge, and then keep the lunge in place while you perform the press. Bring the kettlebell back to the hold that you racked before returning to the standing position.

SQUAT SUMO WITH FRONT AND BACK JUMP

Muscles targeted: glutes, hamstrings, quads, back, core

Sit in a comfortable, neutral position, feet wider than shoulder width apart, holding the kettlebell between your legs.

Bend your knees and pivot upwards from your hips to do a wide squat until your knees are level with the ground. Make sure your back is straight.

Grab your kettlebell with firm grips by the handle using both hands.

Get back to a standing posture and then lift your kettlebell by you, and then letting it hang over your head.

Continue the wide-squat until you return your kettlebell to the ground.

From the squat position, lift off the floor in an explosive jump backwards from the kettlebell.

Place your knees with your knees slightly bent , and return to your wide squat.

Then, you can push off the ground by jumping forward with explosive force to your kettlebell, then come back to a standing posture.

DOUBLE LUNGE OVERHEAD

Muscles to be targeted: shoulders, glutes, core, hamstrings and quads

Place your feet shoulder width apart, with your kettlebell with the rack position.

Reach your arm straight overhead for presses. Make sure your arms are straight and aligned with your elbow, wrist, and shoulder aligned with one another.

Reverse your left leg while performing an inverse lunge.

Return to a standing posture.

Move forward using your left leg while performing an ordinary lunge.

Return to a standing posture.

When you perform the lunge the side that you hold the kettlebell should be on the same side that you are holding it on as your forward-facing knee.

Chapter 13: Kettlebells Beginner's Workout

This workout for beginners is appropriate for male and female those who are considering using kettlebells in order to boost their fitness levels in the beginning or following a lengthy period.

The first thing necessary when doing this exercise is clothes. It is essential to wear loose clothing while working out with kettlebells. Most likely, you'll need shorts or any other clothing which allows you a wide range of motion , especially in the arms and legs. When it comes to shoes kettlebell users tend to train without shoes, giving the user full control. However, If you're concerned about harming your feet by stepping on unfriendly surfaces, then use vibram fiverfingers that can provide you with safety and comfort. In other cases, you could exercise in flat-soled footwear, however, you should avoid expensive unbalanced shoes since you'll require near contact with ground in order to ensure you're in a good balance during your workout.

The Workout

The workout is relatively easy and will require just two exercises, namely kettlebell swings as well as Turkish wears. The workout shouldn't require a lot of time and takes about 20 minutes for completion; A two-minute warm-up prior to the program is suggested along with a one-minute active recovery between each exercise. A 3 to four-minute cool-down will be followed by a 3 - 4 minute cool down session following which the workout will end. Be aware that the focus of the workout should not be on slicing through the exercises at a fast pace Instead, be patient and complete each exercise with complete concentration, making sure your posture is proper.

The exercise routine is explained in the following manner and, even although some people might not find the weights be difficult, the workout becomes a lot more difficult when you add active recovery to it. In addition, starting using light weights is vital for novices as it's the method that is the most important in their case.

Kettlebell swings - four set of each 15 rep.

Men - 16kg.

Women - 8kg.

A kettlebell swing can be a key element of any kettlebell workout when done properly it can create the necessary conditions to perform a vigorous workout which helps build a strong posture by strengthening glutes back, hamstrings, and shoulders muscles. Additionally, it boosts the cardiovascular system. Therefore it is recommended to put a particular concentration on this workout.

The kettlebell's swing trains all the muscles required for a perfect vertical jump but instead of actually doing the leap and transferring the force directly into the kettlebell. The kettlebell will enable you to transfer the force of your leap without putting your body in a state of fatigue when sets and reps increase. It makes kettlebells an excellent exercise to increase your jump level that are both vertical and broad. Furthermore, you'll be able to run faster and complete exercises like deadlifts and squats with the highest potential too.

Use a broad starting position and keep your feet about 1.5 times the length of your shoulders with your toes pointed toward the outwards. Your stance is vital because you'll need to be able to accommodate the kettlebell as it starts in a reverse swing. Additionally, you'll have greater stability in the event that your kettlebell sits close to the upper part of your body.

Then, squat with your spine straight, while still not being vertical. simply keep the body in its normal size. As you lift the weight to squat, then keep your body straight, your shoulders on your back. Keep your head straight when doing this exercise and make certain to look around the room while doing this!

Begin to move the kettlebell while squatting with your hips pushed back till your lower back and groin are free from the kettlebell. You can now flick the kettlebell into your thighs to create some speed, while making sure that your arms don't move throughout the entire process This is the only moment when your arms are used to move the weight.

As you gain momentum, you should sense your forearms exerting pressure on your groin. If this is the case, then you're doing it correctly. The kettlebell should now be extended right behind you. And when it is at its highest decline, do a squat and thrust your pelvis in a direction of the forward, while at the same time.

The final step will lead to a tightened back which results in forward movement by the kettlebell. Try your best to lift it as far as you can on your chest. If you can, lifting it up towards your head is permissible, however for beginners the chest height is sufficient of a goal.

To continue repeating the exercise Let the kettlebell drop back to the starting position, making sure the kettlebell remains within reach of your arms throughout the entire time. When the kettlebell falls then you'll have to sit down and repeat the entire exercise over and over.

When performing an exercise, keep in mind that the goal of the exercise isn't your arms, and arms should not be employed to lift the weight. Your primary focus should be on your glutes, shoulders, back and the hamstrings.

Turkish Getups 4 sets, 30 seconds each for each set.

Men - 8kg.

Women - 4kg.

You should switch hands holding the bell in between reps.

It is believed that the Turkish Getup is a great exercise for building strong shoulder muscles as well as general conditioning of the body. It is an essential exercise for wrestlers, particularly MMA combatants, BJJ and other athletes who are primarily focused on combat in ground and standing positions. The entire set of moves is a freestyle exercise that targets the quads, core and calves as well as shoulders. When when combined with the kettlebell, like in the present case it can make for a high-intensity exercise.

Begin by lying on your back straight on the floor, with your back to the ceiling or the sky. Lift the kettlebell gently and put it approximately 12 - 15 inches in front of your right arm.

Move to the left side, so that you are facing the kettlebell. Hold the kettlebell using both your arms when they are bent in a position. Avoid putting more pressure on one of your arms because this could cause damage to the shoulder.

Reverse into the straight lying posture while making sure you hold a full control over the kettlebell.

Slowlyrelease the kettlebell's grip with your left hand, and do a bench press on the kettlebell using hands on your left. Also ensure that both arms are at 90 degrees from the floor and your elbows lock. Make sure to keep the kettlebell at this angle until a step instructs you to do so.

Then, bend your right knee until enough space is created to allow the right knee to be firmly placed upon the floor.

Lift your right shoulder off the floor like you're performing a twisting abdominal crunch. Now, hold the body's weight with the opposite elbow.

Make a sudden change in your posture from your elbow to your left hand, however, make sure you keep the hand bent open to avoid damage.

Lift the butt and the extended leg off of the floor. make use of the strength from your hand and right leg to bring your left leg further away from your body. Make sure you are balanced by keeping your knee and toes on the floor.

Hold the kettlebell in the proper position on your bearing arm.

In reverse, return to the position you started from.

While it may appear as if the workout is slow and slow, it should be done in one swift exercise with your eyes firmly upon the kettlebell.

Active Recovery:

This can be a light anaerobic activities like dynamic stretching, stationary biking, jogging etc. Active recovery can help improve your blood flow throughout your body, which results in greater oxygen flow to the muscle cells. This will also clean the lactic acid, which will help enhance the muscle's recovery. This exercise has another purpose that is to assist the heart pump blood. Simply resting between sets can make it difficult for the heart to pump blood, however this particular workout will improve the efficiency of the process.

Kettlebell Beginner's Regimen

Warm-up is best done by using treadmills, stationary bikes or skipping rope. The duration for each warm-up is five minutes.

Guidelines for weights of males and females have to be followed.

The warmup must be completed in 5 minutes on the exercise on a treadmill or a jump rope.

The program below provides an entire week of kettlebell exercises designed for those who are new to kettlebells. The purpose of the program is to help you exercise 3 times per week over six weeks. You'll be able to measure your performance by with the table below.

Complete the column for weights with the weights that you employed for the exercise. You should mark each rep in the column after they've been executed successfully. If you're unable to complete a small portion in the workout, note how many reps.

Monday's Workout

Weight 15 reps 15 reps 15 reps 15 reps 15 reps

Swing

30-second weight loss secs 30 secs

Turkish lookup

Wednesday's Workout

Weight 15 reps , 15 reps, 15 reps, 15 reps 15 reps

Swing

The weight 30 seconds 30 secs secs 30 secs

Turkish lookup

Friday's Workout

Weight 15 reps 15 reps 15 reps 15 reps 15 reps

Swing

30-second weight loss secs 30 secs

Turkish lookup

Chapter 14: Guidelines for Structured Workouts

Each session must include three of the essential moves.

Kettlebell Swings

Turkish Getups

Squat and Press

Note: I usually utilize the kettlebell swing for an end to my exercise. Turkish workouts are great with a back or chest exercise day since they're not as strenuous as any of the two workouts for your legs.

Workout Frequency

It's all down to your own personal goals. A minimum of two 30-minute sessions focused on compound movements are effective. My ideal range for me personally is 3-4 sessions per week, with every session focusing to back, legs, or chest (I don't separate abs, as it is a part of each session due to the nature of compound of the exercises.)

If you're looking for a minimal training, and you want you can do to get the most from the least amount of effort:

Day 1:

KB Squat and Press 4 sets of 15 reps

KB Swing3 sets 30 reps

Burpees1 set, 50 reps

Day 2

KB Turkish Getups 3 sets with 10 reps

KB Renegade Row (with push up) 3 sets of 15 reps

3 sets of pull-ups x max reps

A model of a 4-day week workout is below (generally what I do.)

Monday: Legs

KB Squat and Press 4 sets of 15 reps

KB Lunges3 sets, x 20 repetitions (10 each side)

KB Swing3 sets 30 reps

Tuesday The Chest

KB Swissball Press 3 sets of 15 reps

KB Turkish Getups 3 sets with 10 reps

Tricep Dips 3 sets x 15 reps

Wednesday: Back

KB Renegade Row 3 sets 15 reps

3 sets of pull-ups x max reps

KB Swing3 30 reps

Wednesday: KB Cardio

KB snatchs 1 set x 100 reps

Burpees1 set of 50 Burpees

Best Time of the Day to Train

What you do for exercise will usually depend on your personal circumstances like work, children access, etc. I am a huge advocate of morning workouts in the early morning when you can due to the following reasons:

It's a fantastic way to begin your day and provides a long-lasting energy an energy boost throughout the day.

You can exercise at a speedy pace if you want to

It doesn't alter sleep patterns as late night exercise can.

One of the most important things to consider if do decide to exercise at night, is to have a trusted trainer who can ensure that you don't fall over and set the alarm. You'll require someone to ensure you are accountable.

Whole Foods and Paleo Diets

I do not consider this an eating plan, but rather a conscious choice not to consume the mountains of processed, added-in and preservative-laden junk that we see in the local supermarkets. If you are faced with what you are allowed to eat that you don't like, consider asking yourself: would an ancient caveman be able to recognize the item? Bread chips, pasta and biscuits Cavemen wouldn't know what they are. You've probably heard of the most common Paleo rulesof eating fish, meat as well as fruits, vegetables and nuts. So , I'd like to propose eating Paleo in an easier way by offering a handful of basic meals that you can eat often. Because most of us are likely to eat similar meals every day (such as breakfast cereal, a bowl of cereal breakfast or a sandwich for lunch) It is to simply replace them with better alternatives. The following are the meals that I've consumed about 90% of the time in the last couple of years. They're my preferred meals.

3 Power Breakfasts

Two eggs boiled and some almonds (great for those who are in a hurry or "don't have time to eat morning breakfast".) It boils 12 eggs and add them back to the cartoon to can have healthy and quick meals every day.

Poached/scrambled eggs , the half of an avocado (if I have a long and tiring day ahead or I am worried that I might be attracted to eat junk food during the day, then a more substantial breakfast that is packed with healthy fats is what I preferred method of eating).

Smoothie: A good protein powder. A spoonful peanut butter, and a handful of fruit (I prefer Sunwarrior protein powder because the powder doesn't trigger bloating as Whey, and I'm not a fan of soy.)

There are a few options to choose from Simple and nice. I'd also recommend an iced coffee or black in the event that you have to and at minimum 500ml of water first of the day.

Supplements that work

A top-quality name in fish oils. Make use of www.labdoor.com (Comparison site that actually test products in the lab to determine the best quality.)

Vitamin D supplements should You should aim for 5000 to 10,000IU daily that is more than the majority of supplements offer. If you're not receiving 1 hour or more of sunlight on your face , and an adequate amount of sunlight on your body , chances are that your vitamin D levels aren't optimal, even if they are not.

2 Power Lunch's

Tuna made into a half avocado and served with salad, fresh lemon , cracker pepper and. It's a delicious and versatile dish, and it doesn't require the kitchen in order to prepare it , as it doesn't require heating or cook everything.

Stir-fries like cashew and chicken, with plenty of vegetables (no sweet sauces or rice). I usually twice the size of the portion when I cook dinner and then put the leftovers in Tupperware to eat breakfast the next morning. Some quick tips for a healthy and delicious stir fry include:

Make sure to cook it first, in the skillet before placed on the plate.

The next step is to add the vegetables so that the stir-fry is prevented from becoming sloppy.

Use sesame oil macadamia oil, macadamia oil, or coconut oil. Never vegetable, canola, or olive oil.

There is no need for sweet sauces fresh herbs such as ginger, garlic chilli limes, and soy sauce are all you'll ever require.

The goal is to substitute the calories of rice by using the roasted peanuts or cashews and give the stir-fry a great crunch. You can also make use of the sauce satay (see further below).

A quick method to make satay sauceis boil water in kettlebell , then place a small amount into the middle of the cup. Then, place a spoonful of peanut butter inside the cup. Tilt it until you're submerged in boiling water, which will begin to melt it. Continue whisking the peanut butter to melt until it becomes creamy and then add some soy sauce and you're finished. Simple and delicious.

4 Quick Snacks

Mixing raw nuts with an apple or piece Jerky

A spoonful of peanut butter, and a handful of frozen strawberries

Egg boiled and a handful of mixed nuts

Tiny cans of tuna with a flavor (eat straight from the can using 1 teaspoon.)

They can be used as a substitute meal by its own by increasing the amount of. For nuts , your preferred choice is fresh almonds (approx. 15 almonds depending on your weight.)

4 Tips to Stay Strong after Dinner

Cook your chicken or fish with a healthy portion of asparagus, broccoli, or kale in aluminium foil and a generous drizzle of olive oil, coconut oil or even coconut prior to placing in the oven for 20-30 mins at 200°. Healthy, quick, and easy dishes to wash and you don't need to keep an eye on it while it cooks. You can explore the possibilities of limes, herbs and garlic, which will infuse the food with delicious flavors during cooking.

Stir fry, as it is described in lunches.

Steaming or poaching chicken or fish is easy and nutritious. Make use of one of the standard pots, along with steamer baskets, and then put everything in and place the lid back on and let it sit for 10 minutes. Serve the steamed food on plates and drizzle olive oil or coconut oil and herbs to give your food a distinct flavor (which steaming could eliminate).

George foreman: A good grill that is nonstick. George foreman grill can benefit to grill asparagus and onion prior to putting in fish or chicken.

Additional Tips to give You the Edge

The fact that it's natural doesn't mean you have to take all the fruit you'd like. Limit fruit consumption to just during and after your exercises. This will ensure that the sugar in your bloodstream is utilized and not retained (as as fat.) This is not the case with the berries (blueberries or raspberries blackberries) and can consume whenever you like (within the limits of).

As you've probably noticed, these meals are low in carbs, which means that the body can function effectively making use of fats as its primary energy supply (don't not be shy to indulge in more peanut butter or to cover your food with coconut oil) since there isn't an insulin surge, so your body receives a balanced flow of energy and also feeling fuller for a longer period of time. If you consume more fat, your appetite will begin to settle it's own, not having to endure the blood sugar spike that comes from the breakfast cereal that is sugary, that is followed by a crash at lunch, when you're walking past the donut shop... There is a negative stigma that is associated with fat is not true and I've always thought that if fat could be named energy and made more known, obesity rates would drop.

Try to stay clear of cooked foods whenever you can, because the more alive and enzymatically active food you consume the better your overall digestion health. Your capacity to get nutrients from the food that you consume is directly related to the condition of your digestive tract. A fascinating little experiment that you can do to confirm the above suggestions is to take two seedlings, and then plant the two in separate containers. When they're only a few centimetres above the ground , continue to water one with tap water. The other one is to heat the water to a point of boiling before placing it in the refrigerator to cool. After the water has cooled then make use of it for watering the second seedling. What you'll find is the plant that was microwaved to water will begin to die. If microwaving alters the water's structure so that it is not suitable for plants, what's it doing to us that research haven't yet gotten their hands on? The easiest method I've discovered to incorporate more raw foods in my diet is through smoothies, and eating more raw nuts to help fuel my body.

Drink plenty of water! It's that easy water to your body is like oil to cars. Yes, the car will operate with less oil, but it's going to cause unnecessary wear and tear on the engine, which will decrease its life span. The same effects of dehydration can be felt on your body because kidneys don't function properly to eliminate toxins when the body is forced to preserve it's fluid levels. A drop of just one percent of the body's fluid levels can severely affect both your physical and mental performance. Start your day with an in-depth bath to cleanse your body, make sure you drink at least 500ml cold water within 20 minutes of waking. Most of us be in a slight condition of dehydration because of breathing through the mouth while sleeping, the air conditioning or heating that can dry you out, or because you've been without water for 7-9 hours.

Drinking alcohol: Nobody would like to be the person who is at a party who has their hands empty or having to explain to every person asking why they're not drinking alcohol tonight. It's fine to drink wine, but limit it to a minimum of 2 glasses. If you're planning party or you aren't feeling like letting your hair down, but you want to avoid the harm by drinking vodka and soda, then vodka with a lime wedge is the best choice. Vodka is the simplest spirit for livers to process, and the soda helps keep your body well-hydrated (avoid the sugar) and lime provides an additional health boost that is detoxifying. Finally, try to ensure that you have consumed and digested your food before you drink more than one or two drinks. The reason is that the body is designed to treat alcohol as a poison, and it puts other processes off until it has cleansed the body. The kebab that you ate on your return journey from the nightclub isn't likely to be digested properly and could end up being in the form of fat.

Damage control and cheat days. We all have to blow off steam and have two big pizzas or a family meal of Chinese often. The way to do this is to prep your body an order that your insulin doesn't spike, that causes storage of fat. Here are some tips I have used to reduce the risk of damage during a time when I know that I'll be unwell.

Take a big protein meal and a healthy, fat-rich breakfast to kick off your day. (2-3 eggs, and half an avocado can aid in the balance of insulin).

Take cinnamon before eating an extremely high GI food as it contains substances that boost the sensitivity of insulin to help regulate blood sugar levels.

Almonds before the high GI meal may also help lower the risk of the risk of insulin spikes by as much as 50% because of their fiber content high as well as monosaturated fats. A few handfuls of 10-15 will suffice and will be enough filling to prevent you from getting too much of the pizza.

Drinking freshly squeezed lemons in water is another method to keep your blood sugar levels under control.

The practice of weight training prior to your food intake can help ensure that the food you consume during the next few hours is used to nourish your muscles and not rest on your stomach. It doesn't even have to be gym-specific weight lifting it could simply be doing 50 press-ups or 50 sit-ups in order to activate the Glut-4 (glucose transporter of type 4) which opens the doors for the flow of calories directly into muscle cells. (I strongly recommend reading Tim Ferriss's book 'Four Hour Body', if want to know more about the as well as a myriad of other intriguing cases studies and research).

Also, make sure to drink green tea because numerous studies show its ability to may help in preventing the storage of excess carbs in the body as fat and move them into muscles cells. It also doubles as a fantastic exercise pre-training drink!

Chapter 15: Solutions Common Mistakes to Avoid Kettlebell Exercises

Remedy 1

Before you put your fingers on a kettlebell, it is essential to practice fundamental movements first. The most effective way to accomplish this is to begin by doing a few movements to warm joints. It is also possible to start using light objects such as water bottles to try kettlebell swings particularly if you're an inexperienced. This helps you master the ability to move without putting yourself in danger of injury.

Remedy 2

To be able to effectively and efficiently work with the force that comes from your entire body, it's essential to practice the kettlebell's swings first. This can go a long way in helping you feel power transfer from the lower part and body parts to your upper areas. Keep in mind that your back must be straight and your glutes tense. In time you'll be adept at doing kettlebell exercises with such enthusiasm.

Remedy 3

When you next perform your kettlebell swing attempt to do it at a the movement at a slower, more controlled speed. This is vital in strengthening and stabilizing the muscles in larger groups and reducing the chance of injury. This is why it is vital to keep control of your kettlebell when going downwards, just like it is in the upwards direction. Similar to any other workout the kettlebell swing needs you to control its movements as you move it to the head. Also, make sure your shoulders are in a stable position.

Remedy 4

If you're beginners, it's recommended to begin by setting small goals. Concentrate on doing at least 10 reps prior to you attempt more reps. Once you're comfortable with it, you can introduce a few reps to your workout routine gradually. It is best to discuss with your trainer your issues you may encounter. While it's an excellent alternative to exercise at home, it's crucial to seek out expert advice, especially if you've previously not tried using the kettlebell.

Remedy 5

Flat shoes are best for greater grip on the floor. It is also possible to do the exercises with your feet in. If you eliminate sows, you have the chance of strengthening your foot muscles and ligaments to ensure that you are able to move freely. You can also opt to wear converse shoes that have been found to strengthen the ankles as well as the feet.

Chapter 16: What is Kettlebell Training?

You might be thinking, "What the hell is kettlebells?" Well, these are weights constructed of cast iron and weigh anywhere from 5 pounds to 100 pounds. What makes these kettlebells special is that they're shaped as an actual ball with handles that make it easier for gripping.

Kettlebells were originally from Russia and were popularized throughout the United States only several decades ago. However, in recent years kettlebells are starting to gain popularity due to the abundance of videos, books, and courses about how you can use them. What's the reason for all the excitement regarding it recently? The unique exercise equipment provide users with a different kind of training with weights that targets the most important aspects of being healthy such as cardio endurance, agility, strength, balance and endurance. A lot of people like using kettlebells for its effectiveness in exercising (hey it's just only one piece of equipment for weight lifting) and the challenges it offers.

Using Kettlebells

It is possible to use kettlebells by holding them in either the hands of one hand or both as you perform many different exercises using various moves. In certain cases, you'll need change hands as you move the weight horizontally or vertically and requires you to strengthen your core and strengthen the body using techniques that you've not experienced with weights and resistance exercise. However, in certain cases situations, you'll have to use the strength of your legs and hips for moving the load and, as you do this, you'll get the chance to execute entire body movements that force many of your muscles work in ways that they did not achieve in other exercises for resistance training you've attempted previously.

Of Kettlebells and dumbbells

I'm guessing you're considering that kettlebells nothing more than dumbbells. In a way they're similar to dumbbells since they're weights you can handle with only one hand. But this is the point where they differ. The kettlebells are different in shape as you may not have been aware. Their unique shape offers it a different grip than dumbbells, which dramatically alters how ways that weights interact with muscles.

Yes, handles have a significant impact. If you're using dumbbells the weight's center of gravity is within the palm of your hands, i.e., the palm. With kettlebells, however they are in the outside, and could shift based on the method you use to shift the weight and the way you grip it.

Due to its handles kettlebell exercise makes use of momentum, something that many traditional strength-training movements avoid or regard as unacceptable. The kettlebell also generates centrifugal force that, when combined with momentum, helps in muscles to stabilize and decelerate more effectively than the traditional exercises for resistance do. Training that incorporates multiple directions (multi-directional) that simulates many various movements that are used in real-life situations, such as moving your luggage around so that you can put it in an overhead compartment like an overhead luggage bin on an airplane.

While you can employ dumbbells to increase muscular strength through gentle and controlled movements most of them isolate specific muscles. However, it is possible to utilize kettlebells to build muscle groups in ways dumbbells aren't allowed or shouldn't be usedfor, i.e. by performing full body movements that are intense, vigorous and endurance exercises.

What is the reason behind Kettlebells?

Kettlebell training offers a vast advantages that include:

The primary reason is that it's efficient in strengthening the core strength, balance and endurance. This was confirmed through an 8-week study conducted from the American Council on Exercise. The study found that after having their participants undergo 8 weeks of kettlebell exercise they observed significant improvement in all three factors of health. The most notable improvement they saw was their the strength of the core, which increased by up to 70 percent..

- Improved muscle and agility coordination.

Improved alignment of the body and posture, as many kettlebell exercises offer functional training for various postural muscles.

- Efficiency , because you can work multiple muscles and fitness elements (endurance power, strength, stability as well as strength, balance and cardio) during one session You can cut down on time and get a lot of training.

Increased functional strength overall and increased bone density kettlebell exercises are both weight bearing and functional.

Increased efficiency of other exercises.

Performance improvements in other sports due to improved endurance and strength.

A lower risk of injuries. Rapid stop-and-go movements in sports such as basketball football, tennis, and basketball and many others - place many athletes who aren't well-conditioned at risk of injuries due to the erratic characteristics of deceleration. Since kettlebell exercises aid in training the body to perform eccentric deceleration, among other things and prepare the body for ways that will strengthen it to reduce the risk of injuries during sporting activities.

- A healthier back. Since kettlebell training offers distinct patterns of weight load which aren't offered by conventional weight or resistance training exercises and the muscle groups in the lower back are energized to improve their strength, health and capability to function.

- Simplicity. While you might have to make use of different sizes of weights in your training, you just require one type of apparatus kettlebells. Additionally, the exercises that are performed within a kettlebell-training program are easy and easy.

To be seriously considered

Although kettlebells are an excellent and effective method to achieve a seriously shreddy shape, it's far from 100% perfect. Every training program isn't perfect. Particularly it is difficult for novices. To use a kettlebell with the correct posture, a solid physical foundation - with a solid foundation and strong balance is necessary before using the heavy kettlebell weights. For beginners, it is possible to do the most basic exercises first to build stability and strength, for example rows, squats, and deadlifts.

Another aspect that must be kept in mind is that using kettlebells correctly requires training and practice. The key to successful kettlebell exercises is to use weights which are sufficiently heavy that you'll have to use your hips and legs power to aid the other muscles when moving the weights higher. If you're not trained to make sure you're using proper technique, it's possible to hurt your back. If you're a beginner is best to begin with light weights, then consult with an expert for help in learning how to utilize proper posture or both.

In addition, due to the specific actions involved in lifting weights when training kettlebells The risk of injury are higher than other programs for resistance training. But, the risk are reduced by learning how to perform the exercises correctly. This is why, for more vigorous kettlebell movements proper form is vital.

The most effective way to begin kettlebell training - apart from studying this book and applying the information gleaned from it is to ensure that you're following the correct method of training. It's best to get a second person especially someone who's knowledgeable about kettlebell training to provide feedback on how well you're following good technique. You can begin with the exercises the mirror, or recording yourself so that you can look over your performance at a later time.

Chapter 17: 30- Days of Kettlebell Wod Exercises

The most important thing to complete the kettlebell challenge of 30 days is to find balance. It is important to find an equilibrium in your diet as well as your workout schedule, and rest time. This will keep the body from being able to generate enough energy or getting injured because of fatigue.

For those who are just beginning, it might be necessary to limit your amount of exercise sessions each week to just three. This is so that your body gets enough time to recuperate from the intense exercise. If you're already fit and fit, you can increase the number of sessions per week up to 5 sessions. You can schedule one exercise session per day that fits your schedule.

If you're confident that you are able to complete the workouts that are prescribed as listed in the table below then you can attempt to finish the exercise. The 30-day program suggested in the table below has only one day of rest every seven days. This will result in quicker outcomes in weight loss. It is also a crucial element to losing the weight. It is important to ensure that you have at least 24 hours of get a rest before starting your next workout.

The warm-ups

Before every session prior to each workout, you must warm the muscles you'll utilize first. Since we're always working the muscles of the upper and lower arms it is important to stretch them and strengthen them by using kettlebells with light weights.

Here are some warming up exercises you can do so that you can prepare your muscles to take on your workout ahead:

Name of the Exercise Muscles to Target

Shoulder muscles

Hand Down Spine Shoulders , Triceps and Triceps

Forearm The Elbow Rotation and Lower Arms

Arm Rotation Shoulders

Standing Quadriceps Stretch Quadriceps

Bar Twist Hips

Side lunge Leg muscles

These are just a few exercise routines you could do. It is important to select exercises that help stretch or warm the muscle groups you'll be using throughout the rest of the day.

A 30-day Workout of the Day Exercises

Day # Kettlebell Workout to Work to Target Muscle

1 Kettlebell Reverse Swing and up, hips, shoulders, Gluteus, Legs

2 . Kettlebell Power plank that includes Row Abdominal Muscles Arms, Back

3 Kettlebell Goblet Squat Back Legs, Gluteus Muscles

Four Single Arm Kettlebells Floor Press Arms Chest Core

5 Rest Day

6 Kettlebell High Arms, Pull Shoulders, Gluteus Legs, Muscles

7. Kettlebell The Lunge Press Back Arms, Shoulders, Abdominal Muscles, Gluteus Muscles, Legs

8. Kettlebell Sumo High Legs, Pull Back, Shoulders, and Arms

9 Kettlebell Russian Twist Abdominal Muscles Lower Back

10- Kettlebell Windmill Back Shoulders, Abdominal Muscles, Oblique Muscles and hips

The 11-range One-arm Kettlebell has a Floor Press Chest Triceps, Shoulder

12 Day of Rest Day

13 Side Step Kettlebell Swing Legs Gluteus Muscles Back

14 Kettlebell Pushup Triceps Chest

15 single arm Kettlebell Toss back, shoulders, hips, Gluteus, Legs

16 Kettlebell one-legged deadlift Hamstrings, Gluteus Muscles, Lower Back

17. Kettlebell Pistol the quadriceps squat Calves, Gluteus Muscles, Hamstrings, Shoulders

18. Leg over Floor Press Chest Triceps, Shoulders

19 Rest Day

20 Plyo Kettlebell Pushups Chest, Triceps, Shoulders

21 Kettlebell Rowing Back Alternate Renegade Arms, Shoulders, Core Legs, Hips

22 Front Squats with two Kettlebells Quadriceps and Gluteus Muscles

23 Kettlebell Pushups with Chest, Row Back, Arms

24 Kettlebell Half-Get Up Arms, Abdominal Muscles Back

25, Kettlebell, Figure 8, Arms Back, Abdominal Muscles

26 Day of Rest Day

27 single arm Kettlebell split Jerk Back Chest, Shoulders, Legs, and Chest

28 Kettlebell Two Arms Military Press Back Arms, Shoulders

29 Kettlebell Clean Butt, Legs, Back

30 Kettlebell Dead lift Legs Gluteus Muscles Arms back, Abdominal Muscles

In the above workouts the recommended 8-10 reps with a 16kg kettlebell designed for men. If you find that 16kg is too difficult for certain exercises, like windmills and get-ups, you can use the 12kg kettlebell. Start working your way upwards on the weight ladder until 10 reps are too easy for you.

Women who are just beginning should begin with a kettlebells of 6 to 10 kilograms. They should begin with eight reps. Instead of increasing the weights, however women who are only looking to lose weight should boost the amount of reps.

Integrating the Kettlebell WOD into your CrossFit routine

After you have completed 8-10 reps of the Kettlebell Workout You should then complete 10 pushups. It is important to try to complete the exercise as quickly that you are able to. The recommended time is five rounds of this exercise pair on your days of exercise. It is possible to have a minute to rest between sets. You can also switch the pushups into other calisthenics workouts.

In order to make the exercise more difficult For more challenge, you could repeat identical exercises the next month. But this time, you'll be recording the amount of time it took you to complete the 5 rounds. Then, you can repeat the exercise the next month and try to decrease your time needed to complete the exercise.

Conclusion

Kettlebell Kettlebell used as a weight might have been used for a long time however it wasn't until the 1960s when we in the west have even realised the versatility of this piece of equipment is available. In the beginning, it took us nearly 30 years before we finally began using the Kettlebell to use. Since then, this iron marvel has helped thousands of American fitness enthusiasts to achieve impressive increase in strength and strength and some have achieved this strength and retained their toned bodies. Others have developed muscle definition as seen in the old Greek as well as Roman statues.

No matter what your profession whether you are an amateur, professional, or simply an exercise enthusiast the kettlebell is an essential piece of equipment that you can't do without. With this kettlebell and book, you will be equipped with all the tools required to reach the fullest extent. These simple methods are only the beginning of what you could accomplish using kettlebells. Since the weight is derived in areas, you will find plenty of different exercises you can learn, as well as numerous other ones that you can do with it.

Remember that no matter how hard you're working out, you must train intelligently. Make sure to give your muscles' different groups the chance to recover from your workouts, but do not push yourself too hard and most importantly be sure you're in good posture. technique throughout these exercises is right to prevent injuries. If you are unsure of particular postures or positions take note that there's no shame in seeking assistance from a professional. Security whether at home, in the park, or in the gym, is the most important thing.

www.ingramcontent.com/pod-product-compliance
Lightning Source LLC
Chambersburg PA
CBHW071841080526
44589CB00012B/1077